Features and Management of the Pelvic Cancer Pain

W0105801

Marco Cascella • Arturo Cuomo
Daniela Viscardi

Features and Management of the Pelvic Cancer Pain

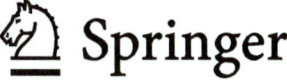 Springer

Marco Cascella
Fondazione G. Pascale
National Cancer Institute
Naples, Italy

Arturo Cuomo
Fondazione G. Pascale
National Cancer Institute
Naples, Italy

Daniela Viscardi
Department Clinical Neurosc,
    Anesth Pharmacol
University "Federico II" Naples
Naples, Italy

ISBN 978-3-319-33586-5   ISBN 978-3-319-33587-2   (eBook)
DOI 10.1007/978-3-319-33587-2

Library of Congress Control Number: 2016944494

Printed on acid-free paper

This Springer imprint is published by Springer Nature
The registered company is Springer International Publishing AG Switzerland

Foreword

For many years, the main objective of cancer treatment has been quantity of life. Only in the last decade, it has been fully understood that based on the patient's point of view, the quality of life has to be considered as a fundamental end point of therapy. There is no doubt that pain is the symptom that has the most important impact on quality of life.

Pelvic pain, due to the frequent neurologic component and the involvement of several organs and functions included in the pelvis, is the determinant of the worsening of quality of life in patients affected with urological and gynecological cancers. Also the understanding that cancer pain care requires a multidisciplinary approach is a recent concept. Oncologists, gynecologists, and urologists involved in this treatment are often unaware of all the possible treatments available in order to control pelvic cancer pain. This publication, I believe, is ideal for those who understand the value of the mutidisciplinary approach of pain and can add to the knowledge a practical guidance on how to include in the clinical practice this approach.

Rome

S. Pignata
Department of Urology and Gynecology
National Cancer Institute
Naples, Italy

Preface

Hoc opus, hic labor est

Publio Virgilio Marone, Eneide, VI, 129

This book does not intend to be a manual on a subject that is moreover very complex and difficult to talk about. It has been designed in order to provide a practical guide, which could be easily used in the daily clinical practice on the management of pelvic pain with neoplastic genesis. On account of this, the book's chapters examine step by step all the more meaningful and critical aspects through a consequential progression. Additionally, at the end of each chapter, or paragraph, we have summarized the "practical suggestions," including recommended dosages and treatment strategies, with particular attention to side effects and possible complications. All topics refer to current literature, recent guidelines, and recommendations on the subject.

The discussion is divided into two parts: *Features and assessment* and *Treatments*. The features of pelvic pain in different cancer diseases and the pain assessment tools are two highly relevant basic themes on the matter. Several studies highlighted that two serious problems of healthcare professionals are the lack of knowledge about pain and the poor pain assessment.

A special issue concerns the pharmacological therapy. Analgesics, particularly opioids, are the mainstay of cancer pain treatment. Indeed, about 85 and 90 % of patients with advanced cancer can have their pain well controlled with the use of analgesic drugs and adjuvants, which usually can be taken orally. Nevertheless, failure in controlling cancer pain with pharmacological management calls for employing multimodal management and invasive techniques, implementing the step 4 of the World Health Organization's three-step ladder. This issue also concerns pelvic cancer pain. By virtue of which, in this book, specific chapters concern the non-pharmacological approaches to cancer pelvic pain, including palliative radiotherapy, central neuraxial blocks, neurolytic sympathetic plexus blocks for pelvic visceral pain, and minimally invasive palliative procedures.

We also dedicated particular attention to the breakthrough cancer pain, "trying" to explain the clinical features and providing some suggestions for its management. Breakthrough cancer pain is a challenge in pain management. Our special interest is based on the evidence in the clinical experience of a high number of patients with cancer pelvic diseases who have to deal with this serious problem, especially those with pelvic bone lesions.

The emotional and behavioral changes are to be taken into account in both noncancer and cancer disease management. Pain significantly influences patients' quality of life and their psychological vulnerability, so specific chapters are spent on psychological and behavioral approaches to cancer pain management, and the role of palliative care team is also addressed. Many lines of evidence underline the effective role of psychological, behavioral, and rehabilitation approaches to cancer-related pain; moreover, when no cure of the cancer disease can be expected, pain management becomes an important component of the palliative care setting.

Because diagnostic and therapeutic approaches are common to more properly pelvic diseases, we thought it useful to include clinical features of tumors, such as anal cancer, which are classified among the diseases of the perineum.

This work is the result of our experience "in the pain"; thus, it is dedicated to all those who ask us for an answer, namely all patients who have been under our care for all these years: how much have we learned from them!

Naples, Italy

Marco Cascella
Arturo Cuomo
Daniela Viscardi

Acknowledgments

We are especially grateful to friends and colleagues whose inspiration was central to the writing of this book. In particular, we acknowledge: M.R. Muzio, Asl NA 3 SUD, Torre del Greco, Napoli; F. Fiore, Istituto Nazionale Tumori, Napoli; Ruben Iskandaryan, Russian National Research Medical University; C.A. Forte, Istituto Nazionale Tumori, Napoli; S. Longo, AOU Federico II, Napoli; D. Carbone, PO Umberto I, Nocera Inferiore, Salerno; C. Romano, Istituto Nazionale Tumori, Napoli; G. M. Romano, Istituto Nazionale Tumori, Napoli; R. Accardo, Istituto Nazionale Tumori, Napoli; V. Borzillo, Istituto Nazionale Tumori, Napoli; G. Esposito, Istituto Nazionale Tumori, Napoli.

A special thanks to Andrea Cascella, our personal proofreader. Yet, Sabina, Laura, Vincenzo, Giangi, and Matteo Cascella; Anna Maria Cerbone; Giovanna Russo, Simone Viscardi, and Vincenzo Moliterno; and Cristina Romano for investing their time to support our ambitious objective.

Contents

Abbreviations

ASRA	American Society of Regional Anesthesia and Pain Medicine
BIPN	Bortezomib-induced peripheral neuropathy
BPI	Brief Pain Inventory
BPI-SF	Brief Pain Inventory-Short Form
BPs	Bisphosphonates
BTcP	Breakthrough cancer pain
CBR2	Cannabinoid Receptor-2
cGy	CentiGray
CIPN	Chemotherapy-induced peripheral neuropathy
CNS	Central nervous system
COMT	Catecholamine-O-methyltransferase
CPSP	Chronic postsurgical pain
CRT	Conformal radiotherapy
DNIC	Diffuse noxious inhibitory control
DRG	Dorsal root ganglia
DSF-KJ	The German pain questionnaire for children and adolescents
EAPC	European Association for Palliative Care
EBRT	External beam radiotherapy treatment
ECT	Electrochemotherapy
EORTC	European Organization for Research and Treatment of Cancer
ESMO	European Society of Clinical Oncology
G	Gauge
GABA	Gamma-Amino Butyric Acid
GSH	Glutathione
Gy	Gray

IASP	International Association for the Study of Pain
ICU	Intensive care unit
IDD	Intrathecal drug delivery
IHPB	Inferior Hypogastric Plexus Block
IMRT	Intensity-modulated radiotherapy
IOPS	The Italian Oncologic Pain Survey
IRE	Irreversible electroporation
L5	5th lumbar vertebra
LINAC	Linear accelerators
LITT	Laser-induced interstitial thermotherapy
MIPPs	Minimally invasive palliative procedures
NCI-CTC	National Cancer Institute-Common Toxicity Criteria.
NLP	Neoplastic lumbosacral plexopathy
NMDA	N-Methyl-D-Aspartate
NRS	Numerical rating scale
NSAIDs	Nonsteroidal anti-inflammatory drugs
PACC	Polyanalgesic Consensus Committee
PCA	Patient-controlled analgesia
PMI	The Pain Management Index
PNS	Peripheral Neuropathy Scale
PPS	Palliative Performance Scale
PRD	Pelvic radiation disease
PTM	Personal therapy manager
QLQ-CIPN20	CIPN-specific quality-of-life questionnaire
QoL	Quality of life
RANKL	Receptor activator of nuclear factor kappa-B ligand
RFA	Radiofrequency ablation
ROOs	Rapid onset opioids
RT	Radiation Therapy
S1	1st sacral
SBRT	Stereotactic radiotherapy
SHPB	Superior Hypogastric Plexus Block
SNRI	Serotonin norepinephrine reuptake inhibitors
SRS	Stereotactic radiosurgery

SSRI	Selective serotonin reuptake inhibitors
TOPS	Treatment Outcomes of Pain Survey
VAS	Visual analogue scale
VMAT	Volumetric modulated arc therapy
VRS	Verbal rating scale
WHO	World Health Organization
WHYMPI	The West Haven-Yale Multidimensional Pain Inventory

Introduction

In pelvic diseases, pain is a common and debilitating symptom which has variable etiology. It can occur suddenly, sharply, and briefly (acute pelvic pain) or over the long term (chronic pelvic pain). Acute pelvic pain is a discomfort in the lower abdomen below the umbilicus of less than 3 months' duration [1]. It originates in reproductive or nonreproductive organs, and the differential diagnosis includes gynecologic, urologic, musculoskeletal, gastrointestinal, vascular, and metabolic disorders [2] (Table 1).

On the other hand, chronic pelvic pain refers to any constant or intermittent pelvic pain. Although it is defined in different ways, the most commonly used definitions refer to both the location and the duration of the pain. In 1994, Campbell and Collett stated that chronic pelvic pain is a recurrent or constant pain in the lower abdominal region, which has lasted for at least 6 months [3]. We can use a similar definition for chronic pelvic cancer pain, assuming that the cause of the chronic painful syndrome is a cancer disease. However, according to recent viewpoints, the distinction between acute and chronic pain not only refers to the duration of the pain but involves its pathophysiology. In all locations, while acute pain occurs in response to tissue injury and then to protect the body against a potentially damaging noxious stimulus, chronic pain could become a disease itself, because of central and peripheral mechanisms of sensitization [4]. Central sensitization can occur when nociceptor inputs trigger a prolonged increase in the excitability and synaptic efficacy of neurons in central nociceptive pathways. This phenomenon of central amplifica-

TABLE I Causes of acute pelvic pain

Pregnancy related	**Non-gynecologic**
Spontaneous abortion	*Gastrointestinal*
Ectopic pregnancy	Appendicitis
Gynecologic: infectious	Gastroenteritis
Endometritis	Diverticulitis
Pelvic Inflammatory	Inflammatory bowel disease
disease	Bowel obstruction
Tubo-ovarian abscesses	Constipation
Gynecologic: noninfectious	Adhesions
Dysmenorrhea	*Urinary tract*
Uterine fibroids	Infections (cystitis,
Endometriosis	pyelonephritis)
Mittelschmerz	Nephrolithiasis
Ovarian cyst, rupture,	*Musculoskeletal*
torsion,	Strained tendons, hernia,
Ovarian hemorrhage	infection
Ovarian cancer	*Other* (Aortic dissection/
Ovarian hyperstimulation	aneurysm)
syndrome	

tion of signals involves synaptic plasticity in the spinal cord and neuroplastic changes in different brain regions, including the anterior cingulate cortex, insular cortex, ventrolateral orbitofrontal area, amygdala, striatum, thalamus, hypothalamus, rostral ventromedial medulla, periaqueductal gray, pons (locus coeruleus), red nucleus, and medulla oblongata [5]. Additionally, peripheral sensitization results in spontaneous nociceptor activity, decreased threshold, and increased response to supra-threshold stimuli [6]. The clinical consequence of this complex pathogenetic cascade is post-injury pain hypersensitivity, manifested as a reduction in the threshold (allodynia), an increase in responsiveness and prolonged aftereffects to noxious stimuli (hyperalgesia), and a receptive field expansion that enables input from non-injured tissue to produce pain (secondary hyperalgesia) [7]. In other words, pain hypersensitivity is the effect of the change in the sensory response elicited by nociceptive stimuli or normal inputs, including those that usually evoke innocuous sensations [8].

TABLE 2 Features of chronic pain syndrome

Duration	In chronic pain, the duration parameter is used arbitrarily. Most authors consider ongoing pain lasting longer than 6 months as diagnostic, and others have used 3 months as the minimum criterion. According to recent views, any pain that persists longer than the reasonably expected healing time for the involved tissues should be considered chronic pain
Response to treatment	Unsatisfactory relief with most common analgesic treatments
Psychological and behavioral features	Depressed mood Anxiety Poor-quality or nonrestorative sleep Fatigue Reduced activity and libido Weight loss or anorexia Increased risk for suicide ideation and attempts in adolescents Excessive use of drugs and alcohol Dependent behavior with significantly impaired function at home or work Altered family roles

Because by definition pain is "an unpleasant sensory and emotional experience associated with actual or potential tissue damage, or described in terms of such damage" [9], chronic pain is called maladaptive pain when it has the features of emotional and behavioral changes and becomes a specific syndrome, called chronic pain syndrome (Table 2). The emotional and behavioral changes are to be taken into account in both noncancer and cancer disease management; indeed, as pain significantly influences the quality of life (QoL) of affected individuals, management and treatment of chronic pain syndrome can often be a very difficult task.

In practical terms, chronic pelvic pain can be defined as pain that persists longer than the time of natural healing, located in the pelvis and/or radiating, in rest or activity, and/or influencing daily activities and with the features of emotional and behavioral changes.

TABLE 3 Cause of non-neoplastic chronic pelvic pain

Gynecologic		Urologic	Gastrointestinal	Musculoskeletal	Psychological
Endometriosis	*Residual Ovary Syndrome (ROS)*	Interstitial cystitis	Irritable bowel syndrome	Myofascial pain	Depression
Endosalpingiosis	*Ovarian Remnant Syndrome (ORS)*	Bladder dysfunction	Chronic constipation	Pelvic floor myalgia	Sexual abuse
Adenomyosis	*Ovarian cysts*	Urethral diseases	Diverticular diseases	Nerve entrapment syndrome	Sleep disturbance
Adhesions	*Pelvic Congestion Syndrome*	Chronic urinary infection	Inflammatory bowel diseases	Mechanical low back pain	Psychological stress
Pelvic Inflammatory Disease (PID)	*Pelvic pain in absence of pelvic organs*	Renal stone or urolithiasis	Appendicular diseases	Disc diseases	Substance abuse
Pelvic peritoneal defects (Pockets)	*Post-Hysterectomy CPP*	Radiation cystitis	Meckel's diverticulum	Hernias	
Uterine fibroids	*Adnexal torsion*		Chronic intermittent bowel obstruction		

Chronic pelvic pain is a complex syndrome due to non-neoplastic (Table 3) and neoplastic diseases, especially when the cancer has progressed.

Beyond this convenient distinction between acute and chronic pain, and noncancer and cancer pain, pelvic cancer pain can have a different presentation, depending on the type of injury, the stage of the disease, and the anticancer treatments. It may be the first symptom of the disease (e.g., multiple myeloma) and—if not properly treated—it may trigger a chronic pain syndrome. Contrarily, it may appear in the final stages as severe pain (e.g., frozen pelvis). In both cases, pain management plays a main role in terms of improving QoL and palliation.

References

1. Bhavsar AK, Gelner EJ, Shorma T (2016) Common questions about the evaluation of acute pelvic pain. Am Fam Physician 93(1):41–8
2. Howard FM (ed) (2000) Pelvic pain: diagnosis and management. Lippincott Williams & Wilkins, Philadelphia, PA
3. Campbell F, Collett BJ (1994) Chronic pelvic pain. Br J Anaesth 73(5):571–3
4. Costigan M, Scholz J, Woolf CJ (2009) Neuropathic pain: a maladaptive response of the nervous system to damage. Annu Rev Neurosci 32:1–32. doi:10.1146/annurev.neuro.051508.135531
5. Jaggi AS, Singh N (2011) Role of different brain areas in peripheral nerve injury-induced neuropathic pain. Brain Res 1381:187–201. doi:10.1016/j.brainres.2011.01.002
6. Schaible HG (2006) Peripheral and central mechanisms of pain generation. In: Stein C (ed) Handbook of experimental pharmacology, vol 177. Springer, Heidelberg, pp 3–28
7. Woolf CJ (2011) Central sensitization: implications for the diagnosis and treatment of pain. Pain 152(3 Suppl):S2–S15. doi:10.1016/j.pain.2010.09.030
8. Latremoliere A, Woolf CJ (2009) Central sensitization: a generator of pain hypersensitivity by central neural plasticity. J Pain 10(9):895–926. doi:10.1016/j.jpain.2009.06.012
9. International Association for the Study of Pain (2015) IASP pain terminology 1994. http://www.iasp-pain.org. Accessed Dec 2015

Part I
Features and Assessment

Chapter 1
General Features of Pelvic Cancer Pain

The pelvis contains manifold and complexly innervated structures that are potential sources of pain. As a consequence, in pelvic cancer diseases, several factors cause pain, such as the primary solid tumors of the pelvic organs and other pelvic tissues, the metastatic tumors, or the nodal conglomerates causing mass effect. Thus, the pelvic cancer pain is a clinical condition related to the involvement of viscera, pelvic muscular structures, or neural structures due to primitive tumors, local recurrences, or metastasis. Additionally, pain may also follow the treatments of the pelvic masses, for example, the chemotherapy, the radiotherapy, and the surgery.

Pelvic cancer causes different types of pain. Due to the complex anatomy and neurology of the pelvis, pelvic and perineal cancer pain represents a prototype of three classes of pain, i.e., visceral, neuropathic, and somatic.

Nociceptive pain originates from potentially tissue-damaging stimuli and their activity on neural pathways. There are two types of nociceptive pain, the somatic and the visceral nociceptive pain. In addition, also the neuropathic pain has a significant role to determine the pelvic cancer pain. Because in most cases of pelvic cancer painful syndromes it is difficult to separate among the individual components of pain, clinicians should more precisely refer to the so-called "mixed pain," which is composed of both components, the nociceptive and the neuropathic pain. This clarification has not only

© Springer International Publishing Switzerland 2016

M. Cascella et al., *Features and Management of the Pelvic Cancer Pain*, DOI 10.1007/978-3-319-33587-2_1

doctrinal value but involves specific therapeutic approaches; indeed, mixed pain complicates the processes of diagnosis and treatment [1]. Nevertheless, to simplify, we will describe the different components separately.

The somatic pain in cancer patients is generally related to the nociceptors' stimulation induced by the tumor or by the mass effect; in pelvic neoplasm, this type of pain refers to the soft tissue inflammation or to the bone metastasis. Bone pain seems to depend on the direct nociceptors' stimulation placed in the periosteum, the release of inflammatory mediators, or the increase of the intra-osseous pressure [2]. About the features of somatic pain, it is well localized, stable, constant, and, in case of bone pain, it increases with the movement sure enough frequently the patient could show the site of the lesion directly. Moreover, in somatic pain, autonomic features are less frequent and, about the summation of the painful stimuli, widespread stimulation produces a modest increase in pain.

Visceral pain arises from the direct stimulation of the afferent nerves caused by the tumor infiltration into the viscera and lymph nodes [3]. In pelvic cancers, this type of pain plays a significant — but not the main — role. It correlates with the infiltration, the compression, the extension, or the stretching of the pelvic viscera. It results by the hollow viscus smooth muscles spasms or the solid organs capsule distortion. Pelvic visceral pain may also originate by the inflammation, the chemical irritation, the traction or the twisting of mesentery and by the ischemia or the necrosis, and the encroachment of pelvis and presacral tumors [4]. Unlike the somatic pain, the visceral pain is dull and vague and may be stronger than a pinpoint. It is not well localized and has the characters of pressure, depth, and squeezing. Compared to somatic pain, visceral pain is often associated with autonomic reflexes, like nausea, pallor, vomiting, and restlessness; disturbances and changes in body temperature, blood pressure, and heart rate; and gastrointestinal disturbances. Central mechanisms associated with visceral pain may be also responsible for organ dysfunction, and a widespread stimulation produces a significantly magnified pain.

Visceral pain is more often a referred, or reflective, pain, namely, pain localized not to the site of its cause, but to an area that may be adjacent to or at a distance from such site, or different dermatomal segment of the body [5]. For instance, the scrotum, with its dermatomal innervation from S2 to S4, may be the site of referred pain for the prostate, prostatic urethra, bladder neck, and seminal vesicle [5], while bladder pain is referred to perineal area, and the ureter to the loin, or to the scrotum or groin. This modality of pain manifestation is usually accompanied by hyperalgesia, reflex muscle spasm, deep tenderness, and autonomic hyperactivity. Proposed explanations are the presence of dual innervation of multiple structures, chemical irritation by tumor-mediated analgesic substances, and central convergence of efferent impulses [6]. In somatic pain hyperalgesia, when present, tends to be localized. Conversely, in visceral pain referred cutaneous pain and muscle hyperalgesia are both more frequent.

Nociceptive processing in somatic and visceral pain has both common features and important differences in neurological mechanisms and psychology. Consequently, treatment of both forms of pain is progressively becoming independent [7]. For instance, in management of pelvic cancer pain, neurolytic sympathetic plexus blocks could be a valid approach (although not as first choice) because of their potential effectiveness only on the visceral component of pain.

Neuropathic pain is a complex and chronic disease caused by the somatosensory nervous system damage or pathological condition. It can arise anywhere in the nervous system: in the central nervous system (CNS), in the spinal cord, or in the peripheral nerves. It is attributed to the compression, infiltration, or the nerve damage either by the effects of the treatment or by the tumor invasion. Often the pelvic cancers are particularly aggressive, as they are characterized by an extensive nervous damage and plexus infiltration. In more than 60 % of patients with malignant disease of the pelvic organs, invasion of the nerve trunks and sacrum results in neuropathic pain [8]. This can cause symptomatic sensory loss, causalgia, and deafferentation. The neuropathic pain in pelvic cancers is very intense and difficult to treat, especially after radiation.

Chronic specific or unspecific iatrogenic pain syndromes are clinical conditions caused by potentially curative and/or palliative cancer treatments. Neuropathic pain is the main feature of these treatment-related syndromes, also in pelvis. For instance, lumbosacral plexopathies are well-described painful complications of pelvic radiation, but neuropathic pain can also have a chemo-related component because many of the drugs used during chemotherapy, such as the cisplatin, the taxol, and the vinca alkaloids, may induce a peripheral neurotoxicity and subsequent painful neuropathic syndromes in patients [9] and in animal models [10]. This type of pain is generally described as burning or electrical in nature. Patients with neuropathic pain may report discomfort provoked by a stimulus that does not cause pain normally, for example, the light touch. Moreover, neuropathic pain often may have a corresponding neurological deficit. Yet, a special issue of pelvic neuropathic pain concerns the postsurgical neuropathic syndromes, such as the report painful or nonpainful phantom rectum syndromes. Phantom sensations are almost inevitable sequels to limb amputation; nevertheless, similar phenomena are described after rectum amputation too, for instance, after abdominoperineal resection and ostomy creation. These clinical presentations are not to be underestimated because these sensations are experienced by about two-thirds of patients who underwent abdominoperineal resection [11]. The most common symptoms of phantom rectum are sensations of flatus (phantom flatus) and/or feces (phantom feces). Often these phantom sensations are associated with pain producing the phantom rectum pain syndrome. Patients with painful sensations had statistically significant higher scores regarding pain and lower scores for social function than those without painful sensations [12]. The phantom pain features are described as either pricking or shooting or like hemorrhoids and/or hard stools that would rupture the rectum. In many patients, pain in the perineal area is characterized as stinging and burning, occurring mostly in sitting positions [13].

As previously stated, frequently pain has a mixed etiology in pelvic cancer diseases. Thus, patients with pelvic cancers more frequently show a neuropathic component associated with a visceral or somatic mechanism. Since this, nociceptive-neuropathic cancer pain is due to the combination of the primary injury and the secondary neural effects. For instance, bony metastases not only cause local nociceptive pain but also distant neuropathic pain due to nerve compression. Consequently, the lack of a pure mechanism leads to serious problems in the assessment and the management of the pain syndromes.

Cancer pain can be due to tumor progression and invasion. However, other related pathologies, including nerve damage, operation and invasive diagnostic and therapeutic procedures, toxicities of chemotherapy and radiation, and infection can cause pain in the course of the cancer disease. Furthermore, muscle aches when patients limit their physical activities and diseases that exist with cancer (comorbidity) also concur to cause pain. Yet, clinical conditions, such as fistulas and recurrent infections, can aggravate the pain syndrome.

1.1 Breakthrough Cancer Pain

Breakthrough pain in the cancer population also called breakthrough cancer pain (BTcP) was originally defined as a "transitory increase in pain to greater than moderate intensity which occurs on baseline pain of moderate intensity or less" [14]. This simple and immediate definition does not characterize the overall phenomenology of a common and difficult to manage clinical problem. Indeed, BTcP is a heterogeneous pain condition which can have a significant, negative impact on the QoL of patients and caregivers. BTcP may result in a number of complications: physical, related to reduced activity and movement; psychological, such as anxiety and depression; social, including decreased levels of working and social interaction; and economic, due to increased healthcare costs [15]. Moreover, BTcP is also observed in non-oncological patients [16, 17] and in patients without background pain [18].

Consequently, a variety of definitions for BTcP have been proposed. The original definition has broadened over time to an exacerbation of pain that could be either spontaneous or associated with defined triggers [19]. BTcP was also considered to be a sign of end-of-dose pain, especially in the UK; however, this idea did not gain a general consensus in the medical community because the main features of this type of pain largely differ from pain exacerbations [20].

The key point for an exact definition of BTcP is how to define the "controlled" baseline pain. Thus, the original definition [14] presents a clear limit, as pain intensity should be severe (on a numerical scale 7/10), but the baseline pain could be moderate (on a numerical scale 4–6/10). From a clinical point of view, this gray area of moderate pain is commonly considered as needing a better analgesia. According to Doyle et al., BTcP is a "transitory increase in pain that has a negative effect on function or QoL in patients with *adequately controlled baseline pain* who receive analgesic drug therapy on most days" [21], while other authors considered it as an "episodic flares of pain on a *treated or untreated background pain*" [22] or an "episode of pain occurring on an *unrealistic pain-free background*" [23].

As the consensus on a widely accepted and validated terminology for BTcP is lacking, these definitions will likely continue to evolve.

Whatever the exact definition, practically BTcP is a transient exacerbation of pain that occurs despite well-controlled background pain, by giving around the clock opioid administration able to provide at least mild analgesia [24]. It is distinguishable from background pain by being transient or episodic and breaking through the stable, controlled chronic background pain. About the pain features, it can manifest itself as somatic, visceral, neuropathic, or mixed pain, and baseline pain may have the same classification or a different classification. Patients can have more than one kind of baseline pain and several discrete BTcP syndromes.

BTcP can be spontaneous (or idiopathic BTcP) or incident (or precipitated BTcP). While spontaneous BTcP occurs unexpectedly and cannot be predicted, incident BTcP is related to specific events. Incident BTcP can be subdivided into three categories: volitional, precipitated by a voluntary act (e.g., walking); non-volitional, precipitated by an involuntary act (e.g., coughing); and procedural, related to a therapeutic intervention (e.g., wound dressing).

On the other hand, end-of-dose failure pain is related to declining analgesic levels. This type of pain is an indication that the background treatment should be reassessed and is considered not to be a type of BTcP.

According to the American Pain Foundation, BTcP is observed in 50–90 % of all hospitalized cancer patients, in 89 % of all patients admitted to homes for the elderly and terminal-patient care centers, and in 35 % of all ambulatory care cancer patients [25]. The Italian Oncologic Pain Survey (IOPS) performed in a large sample of cancer patients recruited in different settings demonstrated that 80 % of patients reported that the BTcP had a significant negative impact in everyday life [26].

Consequently, BTcP represents a paramount clinical problem, and its presence is a marker of a generally more severe pain syndrome, also causing an important deterioration of the QoL [27]. It also requires a separate set of strategies from those usually used to assess and manage chronic cancer pain.

In pelvic cancer pain, BTcP becomes a significant topic for pain therapists because several studies showed that patients with bone pain located in the spine, back, and pelvis may be at risk for BTcP resistant to therapy [28].

According to Caraceni, bone pain is the major source of BTcP and is the predominant source of incident pain [29]. Moreover, BTcP was significantly associated with certain cancer pain syndromes, including those due to pelvic lesions. Yet, the same author reported that of the patients with pelvic bone lesions, 78 % experienced BTcP [29]. This incident BTcP requires an accurate assessment of the temporal latency characteristics and duration and persistence of the stimulus, which can occur in very different ways.

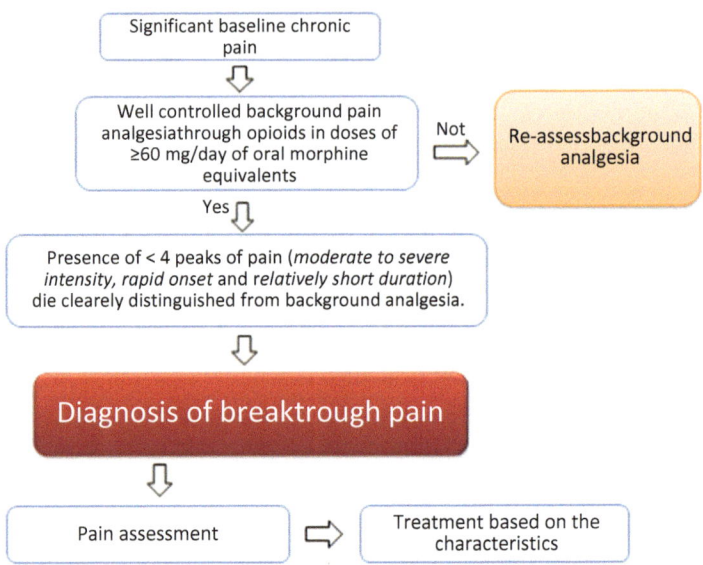

FIGURE 1.1 Algorithms for BTcP diagnosis (Modified by: *Gatti A, Mediati RD, Reale C, Cuomo A,* et al. *Adv Ther 2012; 29(5): 464–72.* —[16]

About the diagnosis of BTcP, there are no internationally agreed standardized criteria. As a consequence, there are published algorithms to assist with diagnosis, but these differ in content [30]. In Fig. 1.1, we report a simplified algorithm for BTcP diagnosis. It is important also the number of peaks of pain, in fact, for BTcP diagnosis episodes must be less than four/day. Moreover, incident-predictable and spontaneous-unpredictable BTcP have similar percentages with a median duration of 60 min, which is shorter in incident-predictable BTcP. Activity was strongly triggering BTcP [24]. Results of the IOPS showed that the majority of patients reported a fast onset of BTcP, which was predictable in about half of patients, while BTcP with a gradual onset was less predictable [26]. Unpredictable BTcP occurred mostly in oncology patients (72.4 %), rather than outpatients and those in palliative care unit [26].

Despite reducing the level of background pain intensity by increasing opioid doses, the number of patients presenting BTcP did not decrease, but a lower number of episodes and a lower intensity of BTcP were obtained, thus improving the general outcome. According to this information, the phenomenon of BTcP should be expected in about 70 % of patients, despite receiving effective regular opioids in doses of ≥60 mg/day of oral morphine equivalents, able to provide acceptable background analgesia with a mild pain intensity for most hours of the day [31]. See Sect. 5.1 for BTcP management.

References

1. Sams T (ed) (2006) ABC's of pain relief and treatment: advances, breakthroughs, and choices. iUniverse, New York
2. Chang HM (1999) Cancer pain management. Med Clin North Am 83(3):711–736, vii
3. Dahl JL (1996) Effective pain management in terminal care. Clin Geriatr Med 12(2):279–300
4. Procacci P, Meresca M (1990) Pathophysiology of visceral pain. In: Lipton S et al (eds) Advances in pain research and therapy, vol 13. Raven, New York, p 123
5. Giamberardino MA, Affaitati G, Costantini R (2006) Referred pain from internal organs. In: Cervero F, Jensen TS (eds) Handbook of clinical neurology. Elsevier, Amsterdam, pp 343–360
6. Stillman MJ (1990) Perineal pain. Diagnosis and management, with particular attention to perineal pain of cancer. In: Foley KM et al (eds) Advances in research and therapy, vol 16. Raven, New York, pp 359–377
7. Sikandar S, Dickenson AH (2012) Visceral pain: the ins and outs, the ups and downs. Curr Opin Support Palliat Care 6(1):17–26. doi:10.1097/SPC.0b013e32834f6ec9
8. Jaeckle KA, Young DF, Foley KM (1985) The natural history of lumbosacral plexopathy in cancer. Neurology 35(1):8–15
9. Casey EB, Jellife AM, Le Quesne PM et al (1973) Vincristine neuropathy. Clinical and electrophysiological observations. Brain 96(1):69–86

10. Weng HR, Cordella JV, Dougherty PM (2003) Changes in sensory processing in the spinal dorsal horn accompany vincristine-induced hyperalgesia and allodynia. Pain 103(1–2):131–138

11. Reategui C, Chiang FF, Rosen L et al (2013) Phantom rectum following abdominoperineal excision for rectal neoplasm: appearance and disappearance. Colorectal Dis 15(10):1309–1312. doi:10.1111/codi.12312

12. Fingren J, Lindholm E, Carlsson E (2013) Perceptions of phantom rectum syndrome and health-related quality of life in patients following abdominoperineal resection for rectal cancer. J Wound Ostomy Continence Nurs 40(3):280–286. doi:10.1097/WON.0b013e31827e8b20

13. Rigor BM Sr (2000) Pelvic cancer pain. J Surg Oncol 75(4):280–300

14. Portenoy RK, Hagen NA (1990) Breakthrough pain: definition, prevalence and characteristics. Pain 41(3):273–281

15. Zeppetella G (2011) Breakthrough pain in cancer patients. Clin Oncol (R Coll Radiol) 23(6):393–398. doi:10.1016/j.clon.2010.12.002

16. Gatti A, Mediati RD, Reale C et al (2012) Breakthrough pain in patients referred to pain clinics: the Italian pain network retrospective study. Adv Ther 29(5):464–472. doi:10.1007/s12325-012-0022-z

17. Portenoy RK, Bennett DS, Rauck R et al (2006) Prevalence and characteristics of breakthrough pain in opioid-treated patients with chronic noncancer pain. J Pain 7(8):583–591

18. Gatti A, Gentili M, Iorno V et al (2013) Beyond the traditional definition of breakthrough pain: an observational study. Adv Ther 300(3):298–305. doi:10.1007/s12325-013-0013-8

19. Davies AN, Dickman A, Reid C et al (2009) The management of cancer-related breakthrough pain: recommendations of a task group of the Science Committee of the Association for Palliative Medicine of Great Britain and Ireland. Eur J Pain 13(4):331–338. doi:10.1016/j.ejpain.2008.06.014

20. Mercadante S, Radbruch L, Caraceni A et al (2002) Episodic (breakthrough) pain: consensus conference of an expert working group of the European Association for Palliative Care. Cancer 94(3):832–839

21. Doyle D, Hanks G, Cherny N, Calman K (eds) (2004) Oxford textbook of palliative medicine. Oxford University Press, Oxford

22. Svendsen KB, Andersen S, Arnason S et al (2005) Breakthrough pain in malignant and non-malignant diseases: a review of prevalence, characteristics and mechanisms. Eur J Pain 9(2):195–206

23. Swanwick M, Haworth M, Lennard RF (2001) The prevalence of episodic pain in cancer: a survey of hospice patients on admission. Palliat Med 15(1):9–18

24. Davies A, Buchanan A, Zeppetella G et al (2013) Breakthrough cancer pain: an observational study of 1000 European oncology patients. J Pain Symptom Manage 46(5):619–628. doi:10.1016/j.jpainsymman.2012.12.009

25. American Pain Foundation (2011) Breakthrough cancer pain: mending the break in the continuum of care. J Pain Palliat Care Pharmacother 25(3):252–264. doi:10.3109/15360288.2011.599920

26. Mercadante S et al (2015) Italian Oncologic Pain Survey (IOPS): a multi-centre Italian study of breakthrough pain performed in different settings. Clin J Pain 31(3):214–221. doi:10.1097/AJP.0000000000000161

27. Portenoy RK, Payne D, Jacobsen P (1999) Breakthrough pain: characteristics and impact in patients with cancer pain. Pain 81(1–2):129–134

28. Hwang SS, Chang VT, Kasimis B (2003) Cancer breakthrough pain characteristics and responses to treatment at a VA medical center. Pain 101(1–2):55–64

29. Caraceni A, Martini C, Zecca E et al; Working Group of an IASP Task Force on Cancer Pain (2004) Breakthrough pain characteristics and syndromes in patients with cancer pain. An international survey. Palliat Med 18(3):177–183

30. Webber K, Davies AN, Cowie MR (2015) Accuracy of a diagnostic algorithm to diagnose breakthrough cancer pain as compared with clinical assessment. J Pain Symptom Manage 50(4):495–500. doi:10.1016/j.jpainsymman.2015.05.006

31. Mercadante S, Marchetti P, Cuomo A et al; IOPS MS study Group (2016) Breakthrough pain and its treatment: critical review and recommendations of IOPS (Italian Oncologic Pain Survey) expert group. Support Care Cancer 24(2):961–968. doi:10.1007/s00520-015-2951-y

Chapter 2
Pelvic Pain in Different Cancer Diseases

The pain may have various characteristics according to the different pelvic neoplastic diseases (Table 2.1). The features and the latency of the symptoms depend on many factors, including the anatomy and innervation of the pelvis and the type of cancer and its progression.

Consequently, in many pelvic cancers, pain is a nonspecific symptom and the patients do not experience pain until the cancer is at later stages. For instance, bone pain and flank pain are symptoms of advanced disease in urothelial tract cancers. Nevertheless, pain from ureter can be typically referred to the groin and glans penis.

In ovarian cancer, pain is both a late manifestation and a symptom difficult to interpret because of the intercommunication of the ovarian and pelvic nerve plexus. Thus, pain from the ovaries is often vague, including pressure in abdomen, pelvis, back or legs, and less frequently painful intercourse.

Contrarily, moderate pain during sexual intercourse is most present in cervical cancer, while pelvic pain, leg pain, and back pain, eventually transmitted to the hypogastrium, are symptoms of advanced disease, with pain prevalence and severity likely to increase as the disease advances [1]. Moreover, lumbosacral plexopathy caused by retroperitoneal lymph node metastases is the most common neurologic complication in patients with advanced cervical cancer [2]. Bone pain caused by bone metastasis is another late manifestation of advanced malignancy. The vertebral bodies are by far the

© Springer International Publishing Switzerland 2016
M. Cascella et al., *Features and Management of the Pelvic Cancer Pain*, DOI 10.1007/978-3-319-33587-2_2

TABLE. 2.1. Pelvic pain in different cancer diseases

Cervical cancer	Moderate pain during sexual intercourse (painful intercourse). Pelvic pain, leg pain, and back pain are symptoms of advanced cervical cancer, with pain prevalence and severity likely to increase as the disease advances
Endometrial cancer	Painful intercourse. Pain in pelvic area. When the cancer disease originates from the fundus of the uterus, pain is most commonly referred to the hypogastrium and elicits a complaint of midline lower abdominal pain
Ovarian cancer	Pelvic pain, often vague, including pressure in abdomen, pelvis, back, or legs. Painful intercourse (less frequent). Pain and symptoms of frozen pelvis in late stages
Urothelial tract cancers	Referred to the groin and glans penis. Bone pain and flank pain are symptoms of advanced disease. Bladder cancer pain can be referred to the perineal area
Prostate cancer	Rarely stranguria. Almost always pain is the first symptoms in case of bone metastasis. Rectal, urethral, suprapubic, and penile pain, as well as back pain and pain in the abdominal area, are late and rare symptoms, associated to the expansion of the tumor within the pelvis
Primary bone cancer	The pain may be quite vague at first but gradually tends to become persistent and more severe over the affected part of the bone

Primary fallopian tube carcinoma	Colicky pain relieved by discharge and abdominal or pelvic vague pain (40 %)
Spinal cord tumors	*Lumbosacral.* Root pain in groin region or sciatic distribution or both *Cauda equine.* Unilateral pain in back and leg becoming bilateral when the tumor is quite large
Rectal cancer	Early stages of rectal cancer may have no symptoms. However, generalized symptoms of rectal cancer may include pain in the rectum and abdominal pain or discomfort. Gas pains, cramps, or a feeling of fullness. Pelvic pain and back pain are late symptoms, usually indicating nerve trunk involvement
Recurrent rectal cancer (cancer that has returned or progressed following initial treatment with surgery, radiation therapy, and/or chemotherapy)	Early symptoms depend on recurrence location, type of primary resection. Refractory and severe pelvic pain is considered a typical finding of local advanced disease
Anal cancer	Moderate persistent or recurring pain, or pressure, in the area around the anus
Bone metastasis (Breast, Kidney, Prostate, Thyroid, Lung)	Bone pain is often the first symptom. The pain often comes and goes at first. It tends to be worse at night and may be relieved by movement. Later on, it can become constant, severe, and may be worse during activity
Multiple myeloma	Pain (e.g., hip pain or back pain) is often the first symptom and can become severe, especially in case of fractures. Normally, the pain tends to be persistent and made worse by movement

most frequently involved bones, followed by the pelvis, ribs, and extremities.

A not well-specified pelvic pain, or pain during intercourse, is often combined with vaginal bleeding (present in 90 % of women diagnosed with endometrial cancer) after menopause or bleeding between periods in endometrial cancer. When the cancer disease originates from the fundus of the uterus, pain is most commonly referred to the hypogastrium and elicits a complaint of midline lower abdominal pain. However, pain in the pelvis is more common in later stages of the disease.

Primary fallopian tube carcinoma is an uncommon tumor accounting for approximately 0.14–1.8 % of female genital malignancies. Although symptoms are not specific, this rare cancer is rarely asymptomatic, in contrast to ovarian cancer. Symptoms include vaginal bleeding or spotting (60 %), colicky pain relieved by discharge, and abdominal or pelvic vague pain (40 %) [3].

In urothelial cancer, patients may be affected by referred pain to the groin and glans penis. Bone pain and flank pain are symptoms of advanced disease. While bladder cancer pain can be also referred to the perineal area, ureter pain can have the lower quadrant and loin, as area of presentation.

Because prostate cancer rarely spreads to vital organs, almost always pain is the first symptom in case of bone metastasis. Rectal, urethral, suprapubic, and penile pain, as well as back pain and pain in the abdominal area, are late and rare symptoms, associated to the expansion of the tumor within the pelvis [4].

The rectal cancer in early stages may have no symptoms. A change in bowel habits, such as diarrhea, constipation, or narrowing of the stool, which lasts for more than a few days, and rectal bleeding (the most common symptom present in about 80 % of individuals with rectal cancer) or blood in the stool, as well as discomfort, gas pains, or a feeling of fullness are more frequently reported. In spite of this, cramping or abdominal/pelvic pain are less frequent (20 %). Pelvic pain and back pain are late symptoms, usually indicating the nerves' involvement. In this advanced stage of the disease, a partial large-bowel obstruction may cause colicky abdominal pain and bloating.

Approximately, one-third of patients with pelvic colorectal cancer recurrence present no symptoms [5]. Early symptoms depend on recurrence location and type of primary resection. Usually, pelvic pain and bowel obstruction from involvement of the small intestine in the pelvic mass are symptoms of recurrence abdominoperineal resection [6]. Refractory and severe pelvic pain is considered a typical finding of local advanced disease because it is a sign of involvement and/or compression of pelvic structures by the mass [7]. According to some authors, the degree of pelvic pain was also used to classify patients with rectal cancer recurrence in order to make a judgment on prognosis [8].

Cancers of the anal canal account for about 1–2 % of all intestinal cancers. They are a set of cancer diseases, including squamous cell carcinoma, adenocarcinoma, melanoma, neuroendocrine tumors, carcinoid tumor, Kaposi sarcoma, leiomyosarcoma, or lymphoma [9]. Squamous cell cancer of anal canal comprises about 75 % of all the anal canal cancers. Its clinical presentation appears in different forms and may be easily confused with a wide range of benign disorders like fissures, hemorrhoids, dermatitis, and anorectal fistulae [10]. Patients typically present with a perianal mass with or without pruritus ani, discharge (50 %), bleeding (45 %), or pain (30 %) [11]. The latter is characterized as moderate, persistent, or recurring pain, or pressure, in the area around the anus. Spread of anal cancer is mainly local and regional. Anal musculature is involved early because the mucosa is very close to the underlying sphincters. Anal canal cancer grows circumferentially, and this feature results in narrowing and stenosis of the anal sphincter. When the sphincter is invaded, the tumor spreads into the ischiorectal fossae, the prostatic urethra, and bladder in men and the vagina in women. Anal cancer may spread via the lymphatic vessels (10–15 %) to the perirectal nodes or at a higher level and to nodes at the bifurcation of the superior rectal artery [10]. All these conditions may involve severe somatic or visceral nociceptive pain, as well as neuropathic pain due to nerves' involvement.

In the recurrent rectal cancer, 29 % of patients may do not exhibit symptoms [12]. However, in symptomatic patients, the pain is the main clinical feature and usually it is a "severe pain," influencing significantly the QoL of the patients.

In primary cancer of pelvis bone, the pain may be quite vague at first tending gradually to become persistent and more severe over the bone-affected part. More often, the pain is the first clinical manifestation of a bone metastasis. This is a significant clinical feature because after lung and liver, the bone is the third most common site for metastases. In several cases of pelvic cancers, pain is the main point to guide the diagnosis. The more appropriate example is prostate cancer pain in which bone metastasis is the main clinical complication and pain is almost always the earliest symptom of the disease, becoming starting point for the diagnosis [13]. Epidemiologic data suggest that among the primitive cancer, prostate (32 %), breast (22 %), kidney (16 %), lung, and thyroid cancers have a high risk of metastatic bone disease [14]. First of all, these metastatic bone lesions are in the spine, followed by the pelvis, especially in the ilium [15]. Osteolytic lesions in the periacetabular regions can lead to pathological fractures, with important functional impairment and severe acute pain [16].

Multiple myeloma is the most common primary bone cancer in adult, accounting for 1 % of all cancers [17]. Although about 20 % of patients have either mild or no symptoms at the time of diagnosis, multiple myeloma bone lesions are the primary cause of bone pain, which is one of the most common symptoms associated with this tumor. In many patients, moreover, pain (e.g., hip pain or back pain) is often the first symptom of the disease. Myeloma cells form masses in the bone marrow that may disrupt the bone structure. They also secrete substances which, increasing the osteoclastic activity, lead to unbalanced bone turnovers and, therefore, to an increase of the risk of fractures. In multiple myeloma, the skeletal site most often affected by the disease is the spine, but the pelvic bone is involved too. Pain is often severe, especially in case of bone fractures, and precipitated by movement (incident pain), without relief with rest; thus, pelvic localizations are very painful and can lead to a stooped posture, reduction of the mobility, and consequently, they have a significant impact on QoL. Limitation of mobility by pain increases the risk of pneumonia, deep venous thrombosis of lower limbs, and decubitus ulcers [18].

In spinal cord tumors, the patients experience severe neuropathic pain with different features depending on the location. While in lumbosacral spinal cord tumors, there is root pain localized in groin region or in the innervation zone of sciatic nerve or in both areas; in cauda equine spinal cord tumors, the pain is unilateral and localized in the back and the leg becoming bilateral when the tumor is quite large.

A clinical condition characterized by intense pain, sensory disturbance, progressive muscle weakness, reflex impairment, leg edema, and disability due to a specific neuropathic mechanism is the neoplastic lumbosacral plexopathy (NLP). It is an infrequent complication associated with advanced cancer disease (pelvic, abdominal, and retroperitoneal tumors) for local or regional progression of the tumor which invades the plexus directly or tracks along the connective tissue or epineurium of nerve trunks. Furthermore, lumbosacral plexopathy can be also a site effect of radiotherapy or a surgical complication (for more details, see also Chap. 3). When the cause is a neoplasm, the plexus involvement occurs most commonly due to intra-abdominal tumor extension (73 % of cases), while less commonly it is caused by the growth of metastases or lymph nodes. A bilateral plexopathy (causing incontinence and impotence) can also occur in patients affected by breast cancer metastases or advanced prostate cancer. The most prevalent types of tumors causing NLP are colorectal tumors (20 %), sarcomas (16 %), breast tumors metastases (11 %), lymphoma (9 %), and cervical tumors (9 %) [19]. The pain is usually constant (exacerbation may occur with prolonged ambulation, or sitting, or with the Valsalva maneuver), dull, aching, or pressure like, but it is rarely burning. It may worsen at night, and patients generally have difficulty finding a comfortable position. Furthermore, the presence of autonomic symptoms is less frequent; one of these, the "hot and dry foot," [20] occurs because of the involvement of the sympathetic components of the plexus. NLP is a very disabling cancer complication, because of the difficulty to treat pain, the sensory loss, and the gait abnormalities, caused, for instance, by the drop of the foot and by the peripheral edema. Malignant psoas syndrome is a subtype of NLP characterized by severe pain due to proximal lumbosacral plexopathy, painful fixed flexion of the ipsilateral hip, and radiologic or pathologic evidence of malignant involvement of the ipsilateral psoas major muscle [21].

A special issue of chronic pelvic pain refers to the so-called frozen pelvis syndrome. This clinical condition is the most extensive form of advanced endometriosis, in which fibrotic nodules and deeply infiltrative endometriosis replace pelvic soft tissues with high-density fibrosis. Consequently, a frozen pelvis causes pain and discomfort due to the nature of the adhesions pulling on other organs. Usual functions such as a bowel movement, emptying the bladder, menstruation, and sex are extremely painful due to the restrictive nature of scarring and altered anatomy. Bowel obstruction, hydronephrosis, hydroureter, bladder dysfunction, and involvement of pelvic nerves are frequently due to partial or incomplete frozen pelvis. Although endometriosis is the main cause, other extensive pelvic disease lead to a frozen pelvis, including infection [22], surgery, benign growths, RT, and malignant growths. Among the cancer diseases, locally advanced neoplastic forms of rectal cancers and recurrence are common causes of frozen pelvis [7]. Malignant growths of the adnexa, such as ovarian carcinoma, may involve an extensive adhesive disease and fibrosis of the reproductive organs and adjacent structures. In contrast, carcinomas of the endometrium and cervix generally do not present with a frozen pelvis.

Symptoms of frozen pelvis depend on the different degrees of pelvic organ involvement and may include painful intercourse or pain associated with sexual activity, severe menstrual cramps, pelvic pain apart from menses, painful bowel movements, bloating, constipation, painful, and frequent urination. Additionally, the involvement of pelvic nerve structures can lead to intractable neuropathic pain.

References

1. Bates M, Mijoya A (2015) A review of patients with advanced cervical cancer presenting to palliative care services at Queen Elizabeth Central Hospital in Blantyre, Malawi. Malawi Med J 27(3):93–95

2. Saphner T, Gallion HH, Van Nagell JR et al (1989) Neurologic complications of cervical cancer. A review of 2261 cases. Cancer 64(5):1147–1151

3. Pectasides D, Pectasides E, Economopoulos T (2006) Fallopian tube carcinoma: a review. Oncologist 11(8):902–912

4. Fitzgibbon DR (2010) Mechanisms, assessment, and diagnosis of pain due to cancer. In: Fishman SM, Ballantyne JC, Rathmell JP (eds) Bonica's management of pain, 4th edn. Lippincott Williams and Wilkins, Philadelphia, PA, p 565

5. Palmer G, Martling A, Cedermark B et al (2007) A population-based study on the management and outcome in patients with locally recurrent rectal cancer. Ann Surg Oncol 14(2):447–454

6. Hogan NM, Joyce MR (2012) Surgical management of locally recurrent rectal cancer. Int J Surg Oncol 2012:464380. doi:10.1155/2012/464380

7. La Torre F, Giuliani G (2016) Clinical presentation and classification. In: Romano GM (ed) Multimodal treatment of recurrent pelvic colorectal cancer. Springer, Heidelberg, p 16

8. Suzuki K, Gunderson LL, Devine RM et al (1995) Intraoperative irradiation after palliative surgery for locally recurrent rectal cancer. Cancer 75(4):939–952

9. Klas JV, Rothenberger DA, Wong WD et al (1999) Malignant tumors of the anal canal: the spectrum of disease, treatment, and outcomes. Cancer 85(8):1686–1693

10. Salati SA, Al Kadi A (2012) Anal cancer — a review. Int J Health Sci (Qassim) 6(2):206–230

11. Abunassar M, Reinders J, Jonker DJ et al (2015) Review of anal cancer patients at the Ottawa hospital. Eur J Surg Oncol 41(5):653–658

12. Tanis PJ, Doeksen A, van Lanschot JJB (2013) Intentionally curative treatment of locally recurrent rectal cancer: a systematic review. Can J Surg 56(2):135–144

13. Bostwick DG, Burke HB, Djakiew D et al (2004) Human prostate cancer risk factors. Cancer 101:2371–2490

14. Aboulafia AJ, Levine AM, Schmidt D et al (2007) Surgical therapy of bone metastases. Semin Oncol 34(3):206–214

15. Picci P, Manfrini M, Fabbri N et al (eds) (2014) Atlas of musculoskeletal tumors and tumorlike lesions. Springer, Heidelberg
16. Müller DA, Capanna R (2015) The surgical treatment of pelvic bone metastases.Adv Orthop 2015:525363.doi:10.1155/2015/525363
17. Nau KC, Lewis WD (2008) Multiple myeloma: diagnosis and treatment. Am Fam Physician 78(7):853–859
18. Edwards CM, Zhuang J, Mundy GR (2008) The pathogenesis of bone disease of multiple myeloma. Bone 42:1007–1013
19. Klimek M, Kosobucki R, Luczynska E et al (2012) Radiotherapy-induced lumbosacral plexopathy in a patient with cervical cancer: a case report and literature review. Contemp Oncol (Pozn) 16(2):194–196
20. Dalmau J, Graus F, Marco M (1989) 'Hot and dry foot' as initial manifestation of neoplastic lumbosacral plexopathy. Neurology 39(6):871–872
21. Agar M, Broadbent A, Chye R (2004) The management of malignant psoas syndrome: case reports and literature review. J Pain Symptom Manage 28(3):282–293
22. Bianchini MA, Bigi E, Repetto P et al (2012) A case of frozen pelvis: primary actinomycosis of urinary bladder in a young boy. J Pediatr Surg 47(12):e9–e11

Chapter 3
Pain Syndromes Associated with Cancer Therapy

Cancer pain is mostly disease related; however, considering that the cancer incidence increases and the survival improves, thanks to the better oncological management, there is an increasing number of patients living with the long-term effects of treatments and potentially curative and/or palliative cancer treatments, including surgery, chemotherapy, and radiotherapy. These could be associated with chronic specific or unspecific iatrogenic pain syndromes, which have often a difficult and specific management especially when they are simultaneous with the cancer-induced pain syndromes.

Aggressive treatments of malignant disease may produce unavoidable toxicities to normal cells, through direct lethal and sublethal damage to the tissues, attenuation of immune and other protective systems, and interference with normal healing. Understanding of mechanisms associated with this complication continues to increase. Unfortunately, there are no effective agents or protocol to prevent toxicity.

The appearance of a new painful condition and/or the clinical variation of a well-known pain syndrome during the progress of the disease are more often connected with cancer recurrence and considered suggestive of cancer development. This gap causes an underestimation of the iatrogenic pain syndromes associated with cancer therapy and the delay in their diagnosis and treatment.

The chronic treatment-related pain syndromes are persistent painful complications of a cancer treatment, in which pain

© Springer International Publishing Switzerland 2016
M. Cascella et al., *Features and Management of the Pelvic Cancer Pain*, DOI 10.1007/978-3-319-33587-2_3

is more commonly due to a neural injury. In some cases, these syndromes occur long after the therapy, so it is difficult to carry out a differential diagnosis between any recurrence of pelvic cancer diseases and a complication of previous therapy.

Neurological evaluation and management of patient scheduled to undergo chemotherapy or radiotherapy should occur as early as possible before their beginning. To maximize outcomes, the oncology team should clearly advise pain specialist on the patient's medical status and the oncology treatment plan. In turn, the care team should delineate and communicate a plan of care for pain management before, during, and after cancer therapy.

3.1   Chemotherapy-induced Peripheral Neuropathy

Chemotherapy may cause both peripheral neurotoxicity, consisting mainly of chemotherapy-induced peripheral neuropathy (CIPN), and central neurotoxicity, ranging from minor cognitive deficits to encephalopathy with dementia or even coma.

In pelvic cancer diseases, the knowledge of the features of CIPN and chemotherapy-related pain syndromes is a paramount issue because many drugs used by oncologists could involve neurotoxicity among their side effects. The occurrence of this "unexpected pain" adds itself to underlying disease's painful symptoms, so the pain becomes extremely difficult to treat.

Park et al. [1] estimated that up to 40 % of cancer survivors may experience permanent symptoms and disability from CIPN, and approximately 20–40 % of patients with cancer who receive neurotoxic chemotherapy (e.g., taxanes, platinums, vinca alkaloids, bortezomib) will develop painful CIPN [2]. Consequently, CIPN is a one of the most common and severe cancer treatment-related adverse effect associated with pain. This therapy-related complication refers to peripheral nerve damage, which develops following the treatment with neurotoxic chemotherapy agents. The vinca alkaloids, platinum compounds, taxanes, epothilones, and eribulin are widely used as adjuvants or primary treatments for ovarian, testicular, breast, colorectal, hematological, and head and neck malignancies [3]. For example, despite bortezomib is a novel agent in treating multiple myeloma, bortezomib-induced peripheral neuropathy (BIPN) is one of the most common, with an incidence of CIPN up to >80 %, and severe toxicities of this drug resulting in dose reduction or drug discontinuation [4]. In multiple myeloma, immunomodulatory drugs, consisting of an antineoplastic class such as thalidomide and its derivatives lenalidomide and pomalidomide, are also used. Neurotoxic adverse effects of thalidomide include peripheral neuropathy and central neurotoxicity (usually sedation and somnolence), and they are known to occur in more than 10 % of patients. The most common toxicity is a predominantly sensory axonal neuropathy, clinically manifested by numbness and paresthesia in the extremities [5, 6].

Little is known about the pathophysiology of CIPN. For instance, animal studies suggest that BIPN probably is the result of moderate pathological changes in Schwann cells and myelin, of the axonal degeneration in all three major primary afferent fibers: $A\beta$, $A\delta$, and C [7], and dorsal root ganglia (DRG) neuron changes [8]. Additionally, the promotion of microtubule polymerization and inhibition of depolymerization leading to inhibition of axonal transport within neurons are involved in taxanes neurotoxicity [9]. However, different underlying mechanisms have been proposed for different classes of anticancer drugs.

Whatever the precise mechanism, neurotoxic chemotherapy agents usually cause a progressive axonal neuropathy, combined or not with DRG neuronal cell body changes, which finally may lead to disabling symptoms and signs. The most common symptoms reported by patients include sensory symptoms of numbness and tingling, followed by burning, shooting, throbbing, and stabbing feelings, felt mainly on hands and feet. Occasionally, CIPN is characterized by severe pain, structuring the painful CIPN, whose management becomes a very hard task. In addition, patients with CIPN may experience motor neuropathy, conditioning rarely the motor nerve function, as motor weakness, autonomic dysfunction, and even cranial nerve involvement may occur [10, 11].

The onset time, the duration, and the features of CIPN symptoms vary significantly between chemotherapeutic agents. Oxaliplatin induces an acute neurotoxicity arising hours to days following its infusion but usually reversible immediately or at 6–8 months after therapy interruption. Many times, the oxaliplatin toxicity persists and advances during the 2–6 months post-therapy provoking a pain growth [11, 12]. Classically, CIPN occurs within 24–72 h following taxane administration and, in most cases, is reversible upon prompt discontinuation of the offending agent [13]. Among taxanes, paclitaxel can induce peripheral neuropathy which generally begins as an acute (within 24–72 hours) and resolvable (within months) pain syndrome [14–16]. BIPN usually occurs within the first 5 cycles of bortezomib and may resolve between 3 and 48 months after the discontinuation of the drug [4]. The severity of the neuropathy induced by thalidomide has been related to the duration of the treatment rather than the cumulative drug dosage, indeed, the incidence of neurotoxicity averaging 75 % after long-term treatment [17].

Generally, CIPN is a temporary manifestation; nevertheless, in a third of cases, it represents a permanent side effect of the chemotherapy treatment employed. Painful CIPN can also persist from months to years after chemotherapy conclusion, leading to significant challenges for cancer survivors because of its negative influence on functional activity and QoL [18]. It is associated with high levels of distress, depression, anxiety, and fatigue, affecting patients' social relationships [19]. Moderate to severe CIPN-associated pain has a deleterious effect on patients' lives causing significant physical limitations during domestic, work, social, and leisure activities [20]. The pain also produces sleep disorder altering the circadian rhythm and increasing the psychological distress.

Diabetes, peripheral vascular disease, nutritional deficiencies, alcoholic and nonalcoholic liver disease, amyloidosis, and HIV are associated with neuronal damage risk [21]. Black race is an independent risk factor for CIPN especially taxane based. African-American women have a threefold increased risk of dose-limiting CIPN than white women when treated with paclitaxel for breast cancer. Actually, poor evidences show that genetic polymorphisms (FGD487, CYP2C8 gene, and Fanconi anemia complementation group) are linked with different developments of CIPN, principally paclitaxel based, and more studies are needed to confirm that [22, 23].

The assessment of extent and severity of CIPN should be implemented with simple, valid, reproducible tools. However, pain assessment alone is probably not the best outcome measurement tool, and a more specific tool should include composite outcomes including the full complexity of CIPN symptoms, such as positive symptoms (pain, paresthesia, and dysesthesia) and negative ones (numbness) [24]. It should involve a combination of:

1. Measures of impairment: nerve conduction studies; light touch using the 10 g monofilament and vibration sense with the Rydel-Seiffer tuning fork tests; Peripheral Neuropathy Scale (PNS); National Cancer Institute-Common Toxicity Criteria (NCI-CTC), etc.
2. Level of activity and participation: Total Neuropathy Score or Calibrated-overall Disability Score.

3. Quality of life: European Organization for Research and Treatment of Cancer (EORTC) 30-item questionnaire for cancer patients (QLQ-C30); EORTC 20 items CIPN-specific quality-of-life questionnaire (QLQ-CIPN20); Brief Pain Inventory (BPI); and Brief Pain Inventory-Short Form (BPI-SF).

4. Pain assessment: physical examination, Visual analogue scale (VAS); Numerical rating scale (NRS); Verbal rating scale (VRS); etc.

Individually, all these tools are deficient to define accurately all the features of CIPN and the pain experience associated, so acceptable validity assessments are often obtained through the correlation among the measures [25].

Frequently, there is a lack of information or an underreporting of CIPN-associated pain. The patients are inadequately knowledgeable about the side effect/condition by the healthcare team before the start of the chemotherapy [26]. CIPN was unexpected; patients do not remember anyone explaining to them the possibility that chemotherapy induces permanent and disabling neuropathy that causes severe pain difficult to manage [27]. The effect of this is a delay in realizing and communicating to the healthcare team about their pain and other symptoms, often exchanged with other medical conditions, and the fear that the clinicians would not believe them. Furthermore, many patients consider CIPN a short-term, temporary, or reversible condition, an expected and accepted consequence of cancer treatments; they give a lower importance to it [28]. Patients underreported their symptoms because they understand that chemotherapy could be reduced or stopped prematurely as a consequence of the CIPN, compromising their improvement of cancer disease and their healing process and survival.

On the other hand, despite patients' report, clinicians often understimate the importance to assess CIPN-associated pain and consequently many patients self-manage their pain [29]. All these conditions, delaying the report of the pain and other CIPN symptoms when the neural damage is severe or irreversible, facilitate the development of a chronic pain syndrome.

Because CIPN is mostly a dose-limiting side effect of the chemotherapy agent, the early detection of CIPN-associated pain has a great importance to prevent the chronic pain syndrome, and the treatment regimen can be rapidly changed to obviate this adverse effect. Unfortunately, there are no strong recommendations for clinical practice regarding established agents to prevent CIPN, other than decreasing the dose or duration of the administration of the cytotoxic agent.

Management of CIPN mainly consists of cumulative dose reduction or lower dose intensities, especially in patients who are at higher risk to develop neurotoxic side effects or in patients who already have neuropathic symptoms due to diabetes mellitus, hereditary neuropathies or earlier treatment with neurotoxic chemotherapy, and then who are more vulnerable for the development of this therapy-related complication.

Data on neuroprotective agents to use for the CIPN prevention are still discussed. Although several nerve growth factors, glutathione, and amifostine hold promise as possible neuroprotective factors, the clinical data on these drugs are still limited [4, 30]. Amifostine has been proposed to prevent taxane-based neuropathy, but it has a poor effectiveness and it increases nausea and vomiting [31]. Several randomized clinical trials showed the protective effects and benefits of glutathione (GSH) against platinum-based neurotoxicity and the use of N-acetylcysteine [32], an antioxidant that increases serum GSH concentrations, induces a reduction in incidence and severity of neuropathy, and improves nerve conduction [33, 34]. On the contrary, GSH is not an effective agent in the prevention of taxane-induced CIPN [35].

The use of nimodipine, a calcium-channel antagonist, in 51 patients with ovarian cancer demonstrated an augmentation of nausea and vomiting and a subsequent poor compliance to the therapy [36].

Several nutraceuticals have shown promise for CIPN prevention caused by selective neurotoxic chemotherapeutic agents. For this purpose, Vitamin E was tested together with cisplatin administration [37], Vitamin B6 with hexamethylmelamine [38], and omega-3 fatty acids seem to be efficient neuroprotective agents for the prophylaxis of paclitaxel-induced peripheral neuropathy [39]. Nutrients and herbal medicines, such as curcumin, chamomile, sweet bee venom, and the combination of Asian herbal medicines, also showed promise as protective agents. However, the data were not strong enough to recommend its use in clinical practice and further investigations in the anti-inflammatory activity and prevention of CIPN are required [40].

Like most neuropathic conditions, post-chemotherapy pain tends to respond poorly to opioids or non-steroidal anti-inflammatory drugs (NSAIDs). The management of post-chemotherapy pain includes many drugs used for the treatment of other common neuropathic pain conditions, such as painful diabetic peripheral neuropathy and post-therapeutic neuralgia. However, because of the different pathophysiology and symptomatology, drug-related clinically meaningful improvement in other painful neuropathic conditions could not be achieved also in painful CIPN. Probably, post-chemotherapy pain could respond to antidepressants, selective serotonin reuptake inhibitors (SSRI) or serotonin–norepinephrine reuptake inhibitors (SNRI), in doses below those at which these drugs act as antidepressants. The American Society of Clinical Oncology Clinical Practice Guideline recommends, for painful CIPN, the use of duloxetine in clinical practice [21], assuming the evidence that several phase III studies showed duloxetine as an effective treatment for painful diabetic neuropathy [41]. In a randomized placebo-controlled trial in patients with CIPN-related pain following paclitaxel or oxaliplatin treatment, the use of duloxetine (60 mg taken orally once daily) compared with placebo for 5 weeks resulted in a greater reduction in pain, and patients who received oxaliplatin experienced more benefit from duloxetine than those who received taxanes [42].

As shown by Durand et al., the SNRI venlafaxine (50 mg 1 h prior oxaliplatin infusion, followed by 37.5 mg b.i.d. for 11 days) has clinical activity against oxaliplatin-induced acute neurosensory toxicity [43]. In contrast, a recent Cochrane on the use of venlafaxine for neuropathic pain in adults underlined that there is no evidence to revise prescribing guidelines to promote its use in neuropathic pain, and although this drug is generally well tolerated, some evidence demonstrated that it could precipitate fatigue, somnolence, nausea, and dizziness in a minority of people [44]. Probably, further studies are needed to verify its effectiveness, also when used in painful CIPN.

Tricyclic antidepressants such as amitriptyline (10 mg/day to start, then dose elevation of 10 mg/week up to 50 mg/day if tolerated) and nortriptyline (100 mg/day) have an intermediate strength of evidence and low benefits on paresthesia or pain; moreover, trials demonstrated that they do not improve QoL [45, 46]. Nonetheless, the rationale to treat patients suffering from CIPN with tricyclic antidepressants is based on the limited options and on their well-known efficacy for other neuropathic pain conditions.

Data about the utilization of lamotrigine are not significant, thus the guideline does not recommend it because of low effectiveness, also in other neuropathies not caused by chemotherapy [47]. There was no indication that levetiracetam was effective in reducing neuropathic pain and it was associated with an increase in adverse events [48]. Other antiepileptic drugs, especially the Gamma-Amino Butyric Acid (GABA) analogues, gabapentin, and pregabalin, are normally used by physicians for painful CIPN because of their established efficacy for other forms of neuropathic pain and the limited CIPN treatment options, such as the use of tricyclic antidepressants. However, a trial ad hoc failed to demonstrate any benefit of using gabapentin to treat symptoms caused by CIPN compared to placebo [49]. Carbamazepine is probably effective in some people with chronic neuropathic pain, so it could be useful to treat pain-related CIPN. Nevertheless, no trial on carbamazepine in patients affected by chronic neuropathic pain was longer than 4 weeks nor used outcomes equivalent to substantial clinical benefit [50].

A single trial supported that a topical gel preparation containing baclofen (10 mg), amitriptyline (40 mg), and ketamine (20 mg) could represent a valid option for patients who have neuropathic pain associated with chemotherapy improving the QoL [51]. Topical capsaicin preparations have also been used efficaciously in peripheral neuropathic pain. Evidence of its effectiveness in CIPN has not yet been established. A promising choice is topical menthol. Menthol, a topical cooling agent, selectively activates TRPM-8 receptors generally upregulated in sensory nerve injury. A phase II clinical trial based on topical 1 % menthol showed that in 83 % of 29 patients with painful CIPN, pain improvement is after 4–6 weeks [52]. Another study revealed a 10 % decrease in 75 % of 27 patients with painful CIPN and 50 % showed over 30 % decrease in self-reported symptoms applying 1 % topical menthol twice daily [53]. Additional studies are needed to evaluate the efficacy and safety of a number of topical therapies.

Overall, no drug can be proposed as a gold standard to prevent or treat CIPN [54], and this side effect is still difficult to prevent and control without resorting to dose reduction or cessation of chemotherapy treatment. Consequently, there is a strong discrepancy between the optimistic results of animal studies and the poor outcomes of clinical trials.

Practical Suggestions

- Considering always during the cancer treatment, the development of chemotherapy pain syndrome
- Analyze the antineoplastic agents used and their neurotoxic effects
- Identify the possible patients' risk factor for increased susceptibility to CIPN
- Assess the painful CIPN with specific tools
- Give adequate information to the patients about chemotherapy adverse effects and give serious attention to their symptoms for the purpose of the early detection of CIPN-associated pain and the prevention of a chronic pain syndrome
- There are no strong recommendations about the use of specific neuroprotective agents
- Reduce cumulative dose and utilize lower dose intensities
- Do not treat painful CIPN with opioids or NSAIDs
- Treat painful CIPN with antidepressants especially (duloxetine 60 mg taken orally once daily) or anticonvulsants (pregabalin and gabapentin) after a discussion with the patients about the limited scientific evidence and potential adverse effects or benefits and cost.
- Considering the use of topical amitriptyline + ketamine + baclofen gel or menthol topical therapy

3.2   Postradiation Pain Syndromes

Radiation therapy (RT) is a treatment of choice in the management of several cancers; in fact, it is used in at least 50 % of cancer patients and plays a critical role in 25 % of cancer cures. In particular, it is involved in the treatment of malignant pelvic tumors, such as endometrial, cervical, rectal, bladder, and anal cancers [55–57], as well as can provide efficient palliation of pain and various symptoms of advanced pelvic cancer diseases (see Chap. 6). However, acute and late onset radiation-induced toxicity is still frequently observed, despite recent improvements in radiation techniques [58]. This is one of the main question and greatest challenge for the pain specialist, by virtue of which several studies on gynecological cancer patients indicate that RT is more associated with long-term sequelae of pain than surgery and chemotherapy [59, 60].

In contrast with the chemotherapy, the radiation protocols typically cause not only acute toxicities, but induce permanent tissue damage that result in lifelong risk for the patient. Unlike chemotherapy, however, radiation damage is anatomically site-specific; toxicity is localized to irradiate tissue volumes [61, 62]. Degree of damage depends on treatment regimen-related factors, which include type of radiation utilized, total dose administered, field size/fractionation, the length of follow-up, the assessment method, the type and stage of cancer, and several other variables [63]. Permanent radiation-induced damage places the patient at continual risk for other sequelae because of the normal physiologic repair mechanism compromised.

Once the radiation-induced toxicity is developed, the management of cancer treatment may be challenging due to the scarce therapeutic options. Therefore, the prevention of radiation-induced toxicity represents a reasonable way to avoid a dramatic drop of the QoL [64, 65].

For this purpose, new highly conformal external beam and brachytherapy techniques have led to important reductions in recurrence and patient morbidity and mortality. The Intensity Modulated Radiation Therapy (IMRT) has a strong potential to reduce both acute and chronic RT toxicities by decreasing the amount of radiation dose delivered to the adjacent normal tissues (the small bowel, bladder, rectum, bone marrow, and other organs at risk) than conventional or conformal radiotherapy (CRT) [66].

Mostly, radiation-related pain is a consequence of insufficiency fractures. The effect of irradiation on bone tissue is not completely understood; however, damage occurs at the bone matrix and at the cellular as well as the vascular level. This may lead to atrophy and further reduction of the functional components of the bony structure, making it more susceptible to insufficiency fractures at weight-bearing areas and then to pain. The bony structures of the pelvis lie in proximity to the uterine cervix; thus, single or multiple fractures are frequent complication of RT for uterine cervical cancer in older women, with a 5-year cumulative prevalence up to 45 % [67]. Irradiation for cervical cancer is not the unique cause of pelvic insufficiency fractures and the impact of irradiation varied by cancer site, as treatment for anal cancer was associated with a higher risk of pelvic fractures, than for cervical cancer, or rectal cancer [68].

Additionally, during RT of tumors in the abdomen or pelvis, the intestine is an important normal tissue at risk, and chronic radiation enteritis and proctitis are usually reported by physicians [69]. Pelvic radiation disease (PRD) refers to gastrointestinal radiation-induced toxicity [70]. It is a major complication of RT and several patient-related risk factors have been identified, including diabetes [71], inflammatory bowel diseases (Crohn's disease and ulcerative colitis) [58], and collagen vascular diseases (scleroderma, systemic lupus erythematous) [72]. Tobacco smoking and a body mass index <18.5 kg/m^2 increase the risk of developing radiation-induced side effects [63]. Early radiation enteropathy occurs within 3 months of radiation therapy and affects the QoL at the time of treatment (acute PRD). The main symptoms, such as nausea/vomiting, diarrhea, and abdominal pain, become manifest during RT, but usually subside once the course of RT is over. Contrarily, chronic PRD occurs more than 3 months after RT and is characterized by malabsorption of nutrients, abnormal propulsion of intestinal contents, and chronic abdominal and/or pelvic pain, the latter due to the bowel stricture, or obstruction, that often require surgical evaluation [63, 73, 74]. It represents a highly important issue for long-term cancer survivors with few therapeutic options and substantial long-term morbidity and mortality [69]. Chronic radiation cystitis after RT for bladder, prostate [75], rectum, or gynecological cancers, as well as dyspareunia and other distressful symptoms after treatment for early cervical cancer, is also reported [76].

Other painful complications of pelvic radiation are lumbosacral plexopathies [77], which are more serious when associated with concomitant chemotherapy; indeed, the effects of radiation correlate with the dose, the technique, and the concomitant use of chemotherapy. The mechanism may connect to localized ischemia and subsequent soft-tissue fibrosis due to microvascular insufficiency. Doses of above 1000 centiGray (cGy) could produce pathologic changes in Schwann cells, endoneural fibroblasts, vascular cells, and perineural cells. Anterior and posterior nervous roots injury has been shown with doses of 3500 Gray (Gy) in rodents. However, combined modality therapy may alter predicted tolerability and potential for late effects [78]. Some studies demonstrated that radiation-induced lumbosacral plexopathy is typical of uterine, cervical, ovarian, rectal, and testicular cancers, as well as in the lymphomas [79]. The most common patients' clinical presentation is the painless weakness in one or both legs. Sensory loss occurs in 50–75 % of patients and it becomes more severe with worsening of motor impairment, which adds to disability significantly. The pain manifests early only in 10 % of patients. It is described like aching, burning, pulling, cramping, or lancinating pain [80].

Generally, the benefits of RT connect with change in pain intensity measured by pain scores and pain relief in cancer patient; only few trials analyze the increase and the worsening of cancer pain. Worsening of symptoms, including pain, has been observed following treatments with hormones in patients with breast and prostate cancers, influencing the subsequent response to hormonal therapy [81]. This phenomenon has been defined as "flare." In radiopharmaceutical trials for the palliation of painful bone metastases, pain flare has been also reported [82, 83]. Palliative radiotherapy has a meaningful impact in the treatment of painful osseous metastases (see Chap. 6). In the Canadian Bone Metastases Trial, pain flare was defined as "a two-point increase in the worst pain score (0–10) compared to baseline with no decrease in analgesic intake, or a 25 % increase in analgesic intake with no decrease in worst pain score" [84]. Pain flare must be distinguished from progression of pain by requiring the worst pain score and analgesic intake return to baseline levels after the increase/flare. According to Loblaw et al. [85], this paradoxical pain complication is common after palliative radiotherapy for bone metastases, in approximately 40 % of patients [86], and the patients receiving single fraction RT may be at higher risk. Re-irradiation for painful pelvic bone metastases causes severe pain flare in about 10 % of patients [87].

The missed assessment of pain and the lacking treatment provoke the development of chronic pain syndrome induced by RT. The exact prevalence of chronic pelvic pain following RT is difficult to estimate, due to the concomitant presence of possible confounding factors, including the progression of the cancer disease, BTcP, the difficulty to assess pain flare, as well as the difficulty to compare because of various methods used to assess and analyze pain in different studies. Consequently, the assessment of acute pain condition, like pain flare, is of paramount importance. Although patient's self-assessment, by recording NRS or VAS values—for instance, before the treatment, daily during the treatment, and for 10 days after the end of radiation treatment—remains the preferred measure of advantage, a structured QoL questionnaire with reference to pain location, timeframes variations, and the correlation with the analgesic intake, could be a more reliable tool for pain assessment after RT [88–90].

Even if the exact mechanism of pain flare is unknown, it may be due to an imbalance between proinflammatory and anti-inflammatory cytokines. Prostaglandins are produced at the metastatic site by both cancer cells and responding immune cells [91]. According to this consideration, it has shown that dexamethasone (8 mg) just before palliative radiotherapy and for 3 consecutive days after treatment—when pain flare incidence is highest—is an effective prophylactic agent in the prevention of radiation-induced pain flare in patient with bone metastases [92]. A recent randomized placebo-controlled, phase III trial showed that two 4 mg dexamethasone tablets taken orally at least 1 h before the start of radiation treatment are able to prevent this complication [93]. In the same way, preemptive methylprednisolone infusion (5 mg/kg) just before initiation of short-course RT and in patients with vertebral metastases during the 2-week follow-up period demonstrated a significant reduction in pain score, incidence, and duration of pain flare, a significant improvement in most of the elements of functional status of the BPI and in the motor status of patients [94].

Recommendations

- Implement accurate physical examination during radiation therapy
- Considering the "pain flare phenomenon" and record pain before the treatment, daily during the treatment, and for 10 days after the end of radiation treatment
- Use new highly conformal radiation techniques to reduce acute and late toxicities
- Evaluate the preemptive therapy with dexamethasone (4 or 8 mg) or methylprednisolone infusion (5 mg/kg) to reduce the "pain flare phenomenon"
- Decrease the total dose administered and the duration of treatment, change the type of radiation utilized and the chemotherapy associated
- Realize adequate follow-up examining all the apparatus that should involve in late RT complications

3.3   Chronic Postsurgical Pain and Postsurgical Pain Syndromes

Chronic postsurgical pain (CPSP) and iatrogenic pain syndromes have been established to be a paramount problem following surgical procedures [95]. Many common interventions such as mastectomy, cesarean section, hysterectomy, amputation, cardiac surgery, hernia repair, cholecystectomy, hip replacement, and thoracotomy are recognized as causes of chronic pain and postsurgical pain syndrome [96, 97].

Several risk factors have been identified for the development of CPSP. They are related to surgery, patient, and concomitant treatments, such as radiotherapy and chemotherapy. All these risk factors can interfere also during pelvic cancer surgery [98].

The risk factors for CPSP can be divided into [95]:

1. **Preoperative factors**: Genetic predisposition; female gender; younger age (adults); obesity; pain, moderate to severe, lasting more than 1 month; inefficient diffuse noxious inhibitory control (DNIC); psychological vulnerability and anxiety; and repeated surgery. Concomitant treatments, such as radiotherapy and chemotherapy, can increase the risk of chronic pain.
2. **Intraoperative factors:** Kind of surgical approach and its risk of nerve injury.
3. **Postoperative factors:** Pain (acute, moderate to severe), psychological vulnerability, anxiety and depression, radiation therapy to area, adjuvant chemotherapy.

Some of these factors, such as genetic predisposition and gender, are not modifiable. In regard to genetic background, it is well recognized that genetic polymorphism influences the metabolism of analgesic drugs, and then the pain perception [99, 100], so it has a big role in causing the CPSP. Actually, the development of this area of study is still inadequate to allow systematic genotype screening to identify populations at risk of developing CPSP. For instance, Zubieta JK et al. [101] showed experimentally that genetic polymorphisms of catecholamine-*O*-methyltransferase (COMT) are associated with altered sensitivity to pain and the melanocortin-1 receptor gene, associated with red hair and fair skin, has been identified as one that confers greater female-specific k-opioid analgesia [102]. Moreover, the polymorphisms of the cytochrome P450 enzymatic pathway influence the metabolism of medications and then of analgesics too [103]. Recent reviews in pain genetics estimate that chronic pain heritability ranges from 30 to 70 but the genes responsible have yet to be identified [104, 105]. The candidate pain genes include genes encoding for ion channels, neurotransmitter enzymes, receptors, transporters, transcription factors, and hormone receptors, such as KCNSI (encoding the s1 subunit of a voltage-dependent potassium channel), CACNG2 (encoding the gamma subunit 2 of a voltage-gated calcium channel), and the P2RX7 gene (encoding the P2X7 purinergic receptor, an ionotropic adenosine-triphosphate-gated receptor that operates purinergic synapses in the CNS) [106–108].

Female population present an incidence of CPSP with a ratio of 2:1 compared with men [95, 98], and older age seems protective, but young surgical patients are more prone to develop CPSP [95, 98]. Psychological (fear, past memories), social (work and life setting), and economic factors play also an important role [109, 110]. A complicated psychosocial personality contributes to amplify and exaggerate the pain experience and induces changes to mood and behavior. Catastrophizing, a tendency to exaggerated pessimism about outcome, predicted phantom pain up to 2 years after amputation [111, 112]. Preoperative anxiety is also correlated with postoperative pain experience, as it seems to predispose to more intense postoperative pain during the first day after surgery [113].

According to the hypothesis which considers an algesic proinflammatory priming necessary for the development of CPSP, several clinical conditions involving modifications of the proinflammatory/anti-inflammatory balance can predispose to the development of CPSP [114]. These clinical conditions include a preexisting pain (not necessarily related to the surgical site), a history of an inflammatory process in the area of surgery, and conditions such as irritable bowel syndrome, fibromyalgia, and Raynaud disease [115, 116].

One of the most fundamental predictive factors of CPSP is the intensity of acute postoperative pain. Indeed, patients suffering intense postoperative pain are more prone than others who develop CPSP [117].

Altered function of endogenous pain modulation should be the reason for the chronic pain syndrome. DNIC refers to an endogenous central pain modulatory pathway which is able to modulate pain signaling at the spinal and supraspinal level and is likely to be under the influence of higher cortical structures. It occurs when response from a painful stimulus is inhibited by another, often spatially distant, noxious stimulus.

Endogenous pain modulatory systems appear to be dysfunctional in many chronic pain conditions such as fibromyalgia, irritable bowel syndrome, and temporomandibular disorder. Impairments and individual difference in descending pain modulation are involved in the development of chronic pain conditions [118, 119].

Intraoperative factor refers to the surgical technique utilized and the risk associated to nerve injury. Invasive procedures, long-lasting surgery, or surgery in a previously injured area, for example, increase the risk of CPSP [120]. Breast and thoracic surgeries, for example, play a role in intraoperative nerve injury through the dissection of intercostobrachial and intercostal nerves, respectively. Many operations do not involve transection of nerve trunks, but nerve injury may occur by stretching or crushing of nerves during tissue retraction or in cutting skin, viscera, fascia, muscles, and joints, all of which are innervated by sensory nerves [121]. However, not only the nerve transection leads to chronic pain [97] but also the duration of surgery influences the development of CPSP, as operations lasting >3 h are associated with an increased risk [122, 123].

A review showed that risk factors of chronic postoperative pain following hysterectomy are preoperative pelvic pain, previous cesarean section, other pain problems, and high intensity of acute postoperative pain. The type of surgery (i.e., abdominal or vaginal hysterectomy) does not influence chronic pain. The author concluded that probably the underlying individual susceptibility to pain is more important than the nerve injury itself for the development of chronic pain after hysterectomy [124].

CPSP is a pain syndrome that occurs after not only extensive but also simple procedures. The criteria for this diagnostic entity were established by the International Association for the Study of Pain (IASP) in 1999 [125]. CPSP develops postoperatively and lasts for at least 2 months in the absence of other causes for pain (e.g., recurrence of malignancy, chronic infection, and so on). Pain continuing from a preexisting disease is not considered as CPSP [126].

Inflammatory pain during surgery occurs because the trauma leads to the release of inflammatory mediators (cytokines, bradykinin, and prostaglandins) from the injured and inflammatory cells at the site of tissue damage. These mediators activate intracellular signaling pathways and the phosphorylation of ion channels and receptors localized at nociceptors' membrane, reducing nociceptors' threshold, and the intensity of the peripheral stimulus needed to activate them. This hypersensitivity results in a reduction of pain threshold at the site of injury (peripheral sensitization) [127]. Nociceptors demonstrate reversible plasticity in response to inflammatory mediators. Nociceptive stimuli are transduced into electrical impulses that are carried to the spinal cord via primary afferent $A\delta$ and C fibers. The secondary afferent neurones are in the dorsal horn of the spinal cord and carry impulses to higher centers via the contralateral spinothalamic and spinoreticular pathways. Central processing of impulses implicates the pain experience. Reversible changes in the properties of the peripheral and central nervous systems produce the increased pain hypersensitivity, characteristic of inflammatory pain [128]. On the other hand, central sensitization refers to a synaptic plasticity in the spinal cord generated by intense noxious stimuli on the spinal cord and by humor signals of the inflamed area [129]. In the dorsal horn neurons, ion channels and receptors increase their function; some hours after tissue injury, there is altered gene transcription that augments the release and action of excitatory transmitters and reduces inhibitory transmitters. All these changes amplify the pain signaling and in a short latency (minutes) increase neuronal excitability that, although fairly long lasting (days), are reversible. After induction of central sensitization, the neurons have more responsiveness to synaptic inputs, including those elicited by innocuous stimuli, exacerbating the pain transmission. The abnormal response involves also the surrounding uninjured tissue (secondary hyperalgesia) [130].

In most affected patients, postsurgical chronic pain refers to a neuropathic pain mechanism, resulting from peripheral nerves or plexus injury [131, 132]. Differentiation of neuropathic from non-neuropathic causes of postsurgical pain is fundamental for the design of effective strategies to prevent and treat the conditions. Major nerves trespass the surgical field of most of the surgical procedures associated with chronic pain, and nerve damage plays an important role, or probably is a prerequisite, for the development of CPSP. Unlike the synaptic plasticity produced by inflammation, lesions to the peripheral nervous system can produce persistent maladaptive plasticity. Damage to the afferent transmission system causes partial or complete sensory loss; however, a paradoxical spontaneous pain, dysesthesia, and hypersensitivity, including allodynia, hyperalgesia, and hyperpathia, appear because of the ectopic pacemaker-like activity of injured nerves and nearby uninjured nerves [133].

Chronic pain syndromes after surgery for pelvic cancer diseases include a variety of well-recognized painful syndromes, such as *lumbosacral plexopathies,* the *phantom rectum*, and the *pelvic floor tension myalgia*.

Postsurgical lumbosacral plexopathies can manifest the features of cancer-related (NLP) or postradiation plexopathies with neuropathic pain and somatic as well as autonomic symptoms. This complication has been reported to be caused by several factors, including direct surgical damage (e.g., wide dissection neighboring the psoas muscle), intraoperative ischemic damage (e.g., prolonged retraction and pressure), postoperative hematoma or abscess, or scar development in the long term. Clinical reports suggest that, among the kind of surgery, gynecological operations through the abdominal approach and renal operations have a higher risk to develop this surgical complication. The clinical presentations depend primarily on the extension of the lesion. In a lumbar plexus lesion, loss of strength in hip flexion, knee extension, and leg adduction occurs. Hypoesthesia compatible with L2–L3–L4 dermatomes is detected in the anterior and internal regions of the hip. In a sacral plexus lesion, on the other hand, loss of strength in hip extension, knee flexion, and dorsal and plantar flexions of the foot are detected. There may also be urinary and/or stool incontinence. Sensory failure is associated with L5 and sacral dermatomes. Moreover, a bilateral lesion can cause incontinence and impotence [134–138].

Phantom rectum pain syndrome occurs in approximately 18 % of patients who undergo the rectum's abdominoperineal resection [139]. Normally, pain occurs within the first week after amputation, but this kind of stump pain may occur at the surgical site also several months or years after the amputation. Although phantom rectum is relatively common, symptoms are usually mild and resolve spontaneously in 50 % of cases in time. However, in some patients, phantom rectum pain can be persistent, and in other patients it can manifest as lancinating, burning, pulsating, crushing, and/or stinging pain. It is most commonly referred to the sacrococcygeal and perianal surgical area and can be exacerbated by movements. Whatever the degree of pain, this bizarre phenomenon has a deleterious effect on patients' daily functionality [140]. The experience of phantom rectum pain can be distressing, as it is quite difficult to define a specific treatment due to the complexity and poor understanding of the condition. Pharmacological approaches may include attempts with antidepressants, muscle relaxants, opioids, or antiepileptic drugs. It is possible to try anesthetic interventions, such as perianal lidocaine injections, epidural analgesia, intrathecal morphine pump, or implanted spinal stimulation, but the results are not guaranteed.

The pelvic floor injury correlated with the pelvic surgery can cause pelvic floor tension myalgia. This pain condition is the main somatic cause of chronic pelvic pain in patients with negative findings on laparoscopy and probably it is linked to dyspareunia, urinary urgency/frequency, interstitial cystitis, vulvodynia, anismus, coccydynia, and generalized pelvic pain [141].

Pelvic floor tension myalgia is characterized by a shortened, hypertonic pelvic floor with myofascial trigger points throughout the musculature. These trigger points generally refer pain to the lower abdomen, suprapubic region, hips, perineum, tailbone, and/or lumbosacral region [141].

These syndromes are an important problem in terms of personal impact and economic implications. While CPSP syndromes are very difficult to treat, more effective is the development of a preventive strategy [141], as well as their early detection and treatment. It may be possible to reduce the risk by giving consideration to surgical approach, pain management, and psychological predisposition.

The surgery should preserve nerve roots and produce minimal tissue inflammation to decrease the incidence of CPSP. Minimally invasive techniques should be used not only in thoracic and cardiac surgeries but also in pelvic cancer surgery. Laparoscopic surgery may reduce the risk of intraoperative nerve damage and pain compared with open surgery [142]. In advanced stages of cervical cancer, minimally invasive surgery can offer ovarian transposition, with intent to prevent actinic castration, without modifying the beginning and the extension of radiotherapy and chemotherapy [143]; extraperitoneal laparoscopy or robotic-assisted laparoscopy is manageable and a comfortable technique [144]. However, other researches are needed to estimate the clinical effectiveness of these approaches for the prevention of CPSP [145].

Pharmacologic management for the prevention of CPSP includes anticonvulsants, NSAIDs, N-Methyl-D-Aspartate (NMDA) receptor antagonists, local anesthesia, and multimodal analgesia.

According to the available literature, perioperative use of gabapentin could be effective in preventing CPSP [146]. However, Chaparro et al. [147] suggested that the use of gabapentin for 3-month postoperative pain is equivalent to placebo. In two studies, postoperative pain scores were significantly lower in the gabapentin group compared with both the ketamine and control groups at 3- and 6-months followup, following hysterectomy and inguinal herniorrhaphy, respectively [148, 149]. These discrepancies between studies are probably the result of the heterogeneity of the surgical populations studied and surgical procedures.

Pregabalin is structurally analog to gabapentin but it has greater analgesic potency and a more favorable pharmacokinetic profile relative to gabapentin. In Chaparro et al.'s [147] systematic review, two studies demonstrated a significant benefit of pregabalin as compared to placebo. In contrast, a new multicenter, randomized, double-blind, placebo-controlled trials analyzing the efficacy and safety of 150 or 300 mg/die in three different surgical models (elective inguinal hernia repair, elective total knee arthroplasty, or total abdominal hysterectomy) showed that there are no significant differences between pregabalin and placebo in regard to pain intensity in each of them [150].

NSAIDs can reduce the incidence and the severity of CPSP, thanks to their anti-inflammatory action. Nevertheless, clinical trials are heterogeneous and differ in type of drug used, follow-up time point, and pain outcomes.

Ketamine is an NMDA receptor antagonist. The NMDA receptor plays a critical role in both the induction and maintenance of central sensitization and pathologic pain [151]. Therefore, ketamine reduces pain and analgesic consumption through the prevention of NMDA-mediated sensitization of spinal cord dorsal horn neurons. It also acts as an analgesic via activation of descending inhibitory monoaminergic pain pathways and prevents opioid-induced hyperalgesia (a paradoxical increased sensitivity to painful stimuli in a patient receiving opioids) and acute opioid tolerance [152]. The majority of trials identified used pre-incisional loading doses of ketamine ranging from 0.15 to 1 mg/kg, plus an intraoperative infusion. Contrarily, in men undergoing radical prostatectomy under general anesthesia preoperatively, low-dose administration of i.v. ketamine did not reveal significant difference among groups in pain incidence, intensity, or morphine consumption when compared with post-incisional administration of ketamine or a saline control condition [153]. The difference of clinical data could be due to the different timings of observation. Indeed, while ketamine showed a weak result 3 months after surgery, a more incisive effect in the decrease of CPSP incidence was found for ketamine 6 months following surgery [147].

For CPSP, local anesthetics may have clinical utility through early interruption of sensory information to the dorsal horn of the spinal cord [154]. Katz and Cohen suggested that the short-term beneficial effects of preventive epidural analgesia on acute postoperative pain and morphine consumption are associated with lower levels of pain disability approximately 3 weeks after major gynecologic surgery by laparotomy. By 6 months after surgery, there were no differences of all the measured outcomes [155].

Multimodal pain regimens tailored to specific surgical procedures should be adopted to prevent CPSP and the development of pain syndrome. The use of different classes of medication to target different peripheral and CNS mechanisms could reduce acute postoperative pain and opioid analgesic requirements postoperatively. Multimodal analgesia has positive preventive effects at 3 months and the other at 1 year following surgery [156, 157].

A recent study demonstrated a reduction in total symptoms in patients with refractory chronic pelvic pain syndrome, who voluntarily decrease medication use, utilizing a protocol, approved by FDA, of pelvic floor myofascial trigger point release with an internal trigger point wand and paradoxical relaxation therapy [158]. Probably, a similar strategy can also be applied to CPSP.

Summarizing, as postsurgical pain syndromes are usually hard to treat, prevention is important. Consequently, improving the management of acute postoperative pain and minimally invasive surgical approaches are the most effective strategies which may prevent CPSP.

Main Messages

- Chronic postsurgical pain represents a significant aspect of chronic pain.
- Preoperative (e.g., radiotherapy), intraoperative, and postoperative factors influence the incidence of CPSP.
- Inflammation and nerve injury are responsible for peripheral and central sensitizations and subsequent development of CPSP.
- Chronic pain syndromes (e.g., postsurgical lumbosacral plexopathies phantom, rectum pain syndrome, and pelvic floor tension myalgia) can occur after surgery for pelvic cancer disease.
- Prevention of CPSP could include: minimally invasive surgical approach and effective management of postoperative pain.
- An accurate early perioperative visit is necessary to select patients with major risk of intense postoperative pain and CPSP.
- A psychological support can reduce preoperative anxiety and stress and then decrease the risk of CPSP.

References

Chemotherapy-Induced Peripheral Neuropathy

1. Park S, Goldstein D, Krishnan AV et al (2013) Chemotherapy-induced peripheral neurotoxicity: a critical analysis. CA Cancer J Clin 63(6):419–437. doi:10.3322/caac.21204
2. Smith EM, Cohen JA, Pett MA et al (2010) The reliability and validity of a modified total neuropathy score-reduced and neuropathic pain severity items when used to measure chemotherapy-induced peripheral neuropathy in patients receiving taxanes and platinums. Cancer Nurs 33(3):173–183

3. Sioka C, Kyritsis AP (2009) Central and peripheral nervous system toxicity of common chemotherapeutic agents. Cancer Chemother Pharmacol 63(5):761–767
4. Fernandes R, Mazzarello S, Majeed H et al (2015) Treatment of taxane acute pain syndrome (TAPS) in cancer patients receiving taxane-based chemotherapy—a systematic review. Support Care Cancer. doi:10.1007/s00520-015-2941-0
5. Plasmati R, Pastorelli F, Cavo M et al (2007) Neuropathy in multiple myeloma treated with thalidomide: a prospective study. Neurology 69(6):573–581
6. Cavaletti G, Beronio A, Reni L et al (2004) Thalidomide sensory neurotoxicity: a clinical and neurophysiologic study. Neurology 62(12):2291–2293
7. Cavaletti G, Gilardini A, Canta A et al (2007) Bortezomib-induced peripheral neurotoxicity: a neurophysiological and pathological study in the rat. Exp Neurol 204(1):317–325
8. Cata JP, Weng HR, Burton AW et al (2007) Quantitative sensory findings in patients with bortezomib-induced pain. J Pain 8(4):296–306
9. Swain SM, Arezzo JC (2008) Neuropathy associated with microtubule inhibitors: diagnosis, incidence, and management. Clin Adv Hematol Oncol 6(6):455–467
10. Argyriou AA, Iconomou G, Kalofonos HP (2008) Bortezomib-induced peripheral neuropathy in multiple myeloma: a comprehensive review of the literature. Blood 112(5):1593–1599
11. Argyriou AA, Bruna J, Marmiroli P et al (2012) Chemotherapy-induced peripheral neurotoxicity (CIPN):an update. Crit Rev Oncol Hematol 82(1):51–77
12. Velasco R, Briani C, Argyriou AA et al (2014) Early predictors of oxaliplatin-induced cumulative neuropathy in colorectal cancer patients. J Neurol Neurosurg Psychiatry 85(4):392–398. doi:10.1136/jnnp-2013-305334
13. Argyriou AA, Koltzenburg M, Polychronopoulos P et al (2008) Peripheral nerve damage associated with administration of taxanes in patients with cancer. Crit Rev Oncol Hematol 66(3):218–228
14. Tanabe Y, Hashimoto K, Shimizu C et al (2013) Paclitaxel-induced peripheral neuropathy in patients receiving adjuvant chemotherapy for breast cancer. Int J Clin Oncol 18(1):132–138. doi:10.1007/s10147-011-0352-x
15. Loprinzi CL, Reeves BN, Dakhil SR et al (2011) Natural history of paclitaxel-associated acute pain syndrome: prospective

cohort study NCCTG N08C1. J Clin Oncol 29(11):1472–1478. doi:10.1200/JCO.2010.33.0308

16. Reeves BN, Dakhil SR, Sloan JA et al (2012) Further data supporting that paclitaxel-associated acute pain syndrome is associated with development of peripheral neuropathy: North Central Cancer Treatment Group trial N08C1. Cancer 118(20):5171–5178. doi:10.1002/cncr.27489

17. Tosi P, Zamagni E, Cellini C et al (2005) Neurological toxicity of long-term (>1 yr) thalidomide therapy in patients with multiple myeloma. Eur J Haematol 74(3):212–216

18. Tanay MA, Armes J, Ream E (2016) The experience of chemotherapy-induced peripheral neuropathy in adult cancer patients: a qualitative thematic synthesis. Eur J Cancer Care. doi:10.1111/ecc.12443

19. Bakitas MA (2007) Background noise: the experience of chemotherapy-induced peripheral neuropathy. Nurs Res 56(5):323–331

20. Mols F, Beijers T, Vreugdenhill G et al (2014) Chemotherapy-induced peripheral neuropathy and its association with quality of life: a systematic review. Support Care Cancer 22(8):2261–2269

21. Hershman DL, Lacchetti C, Dworkin RH et al; American Society of Clinical Oncology (2014) Prevention and management of chemotherapy-induced peripheral neuropathy in survivors of adult cancers: American Society of Clinical Oncology clinical practice guideline. J Clin Oncol 32(18):1941–1967

22. Schneider BP, Li L, Miller K et al (2011) Genetic associations with taxane-induced neuropathy by a genome-wide association study (GWAS) in E5103. J Clin Oncol 29:80s, (suppl; abstr 1000)

23. Speck RM, Sammel MD, Farrar JT et al (2013) Impact of chemotherapy-induced peripheral neuropathy on treatment delivery in non metastatic breast cancer. J Oncol Pract 9(5):e234–e240. doi:10.1200/JOP.2012.000863

24. Poupon L, Kerckhove N, Vein J et al (2015) Minimizing chemotherapy-induced peripheral neuropathy: preclinical and clinical development of new perspectives. Expert Opin Drug Saf 14(8):1269–1282

25. Cavaletti G, Cornblath DR, Merkies IS et al; CI-PeriNomS Group (2013) The chemotherapy-induced peripheral neuropathy outcome measures standardization study: from consensus to the first validity and reliability findings. Ann Oncol 24(2):454–462

26. Tofthagen C (2010) Surviving chemotherapy for colon cancer and living with the consequences. J Palliat Med 13(11): 1389–1391

27. Smith EML, Bakitas MA, Homel P et al (2011) Preliminary assessment of a neuropathic pain treatment and referral algorithm for patients with cancer. J Pain Symptom Manage 42(6):822–838

28. Tofthagen C (2010) Patient perceptions associated with chemotherapy-induced peripheral neuropathy. Clin J Oncol Nurs 14(3):E22–E28

29. Tofthagen C, McAllister RD, McMillan SC (2011) Peripheral neuropathy in patients with colorectal cancer receiving oxaliplatin. Clin J Oncol Nurs 15(2):182–188

30. Hilpert F, Stähle A, Tome O et al (2005) Neuroprotection with amifostine in the first-line treatment of advanced ovarian cancer with carboplatin/paclitaxelbased chemotherapy — a double-blind, placebocontrolled, randomized phase II study from the Arbeitsgemeinschaft Gynakologische Onkologoie (AGO) Ovarian Cancer Study Group. Support Care Cancer 13: 797–805

31. Kanat O, Evrensel T, Baran I et al (2003) Protective effect of amifostine against toxicity of paclitaxel and carboplatin in non-small cell lung cancer: a single center randomized study. Med Oncol 20:237–245

32. Lin PC, Lee MY, Wang WS et al (2006) N-acetylcysteine has neuroprotective effects against oxaliplatin-based adjuvant chemotherapy in colon cancer patients: preliminary data. Support Care Cancer 14:484–487

33. Schmidinger M, Budinsky AC, Wenzel C et al (2000) Glutathione in the prevention of cisplatin induced toxicities. A prospectively randomized pilot trial in patients with head and neck cancer and non small cell lung cancer. Wien Klin Wochenschr 112(14):617–623

34. Cascinu S, Catalano V, Cordella L et al (2002) Neuroprotective effect of reduced glutathione on oxaliplatin-based chemotherapy in advanced colorectal cancer: A randomized, double-blind, placebo controlled trial. J Clin Oncol 20:3478–3483

35. Leal A, Qin R, Atherton P et al (2014) The use of glutathione for prevention of paclitaxel/carboplatin induced peripheral neuropathy: a phase III randomized, double-blind placebo-controlled study. Cancer 120(12):1890–1897. doi:10.1002/cncr.28654

36. Cassidy J, Paul J, Soukop M et al (1998) Clinical trials of nimodipine as a potential neuroprotector in ovarian cancer patients treated with cisplatin. Cancer Chemother Pharmacol 41:161–166

37. Pace A, Giannarelli D, Galiè E et al (2010) Vitamin E neuroprotection for cisplatin neuropathy: a randomized, placebo-controlled trial. Neurology 74:762–766

38. Wiernik PH, Yeap B, Vogl SE et al (1992) Hexamethylmelamine and low or moderate dose cisplatin with or without pyridoxine for treatment of advanced ovarian carcinoma: a study of the Eastern Cooperative Oncology Group. Cancer Invest 10(1):1–9

39. Ghoreishi Z, Esfahani A, Djazayeri A et al (2012) Omega-3 fatty acids are protective against paclitaxel-induced peripheral neuropathy: a randomized double-blind placebo controlled trial. BMC Cancer 12:355

40. Schloss J, Colosimo M, Vitetta L (2015) Herbal Medicines and Chemotherapy Induced Peripheral Neuropathy (CIPN): a Critical Literature Review. Crit Rev Food Sci Nutr. doi:10.1080 /10408398.2014.889081

41. Bril V, England JD, Franklin GM et al (2011) Evidence-based guideline: treatment of painful diabetic neuropathy—report of the American Association of Neuromuscular and Electrodiagnostic Medicine, the American Academy of Neurology, and the American Academy of Physical Medicine and Rehabilitation. Muscle Nerve 43(6):910–917

42. Smith EM, Pang H, Cirrincione C et al; Alliance for Clinical Trials in Oncology (2013) Effect of duloxetine on pain, function, and quality of life among patients with chemotherapy-induced painful peripheral neuropathy: a randomized clinical trial. JAMA 309(13):1359–1367

43. Durand JP, Deplanque G, Montheil V et al (2012) Efficacy of venlafaxine for the prevention and relief of oxaliplatin-induced acute neurotoxicity: results of EFFOX, a randomized, double-blind, placebo-controlled phase III trial. Ann Oncol 23(1): 200–205

44. Gallagher HC, Gallagher RM, Butler M et al (2015) Venlafaxine for neuropathic pain in adults. Cochrane Database Syst Rev 8:CD011091. doi:10.1002/14651858.CD011091.pub2

45. Kautio AL, Haanpää M, Saarto T (2008) Amitriptyline in the treatment of chemotherapy-induced neuropathic symptoms. J Pain Symptom Manage 35(1):31–39

46. Hammack JE, Michalak JC, Loprinzi CL et al (2002) Phase III evaluation of nortriptyline for alleviation of symptoms of cis-platinum-induced peripheral neuropathy. Pain 98(1–2): 195–203

47. Rao RD, Flynn PJ, Sloan JA et al (2008) Efficacy of lamotrigine in the management of chemotherapy-induced peripheral neuropathy: a phase 3 randomized, double-blind, placebo-controlled trial, N01C3. Cancer 112(12):2802–2808

48. Wiffen PJ, Derry S, Moore RA et al (2014) Levetiracetam for neuropathic pain in adults. Cochrane Database Syst Rev 7:CD010943. doi:10.1002/14651858.CD010943.pub2

49. Rao RD, Michalak JC, Sloan JA et al; North Central Cancer Treatment Group (2007) Efficacy of gabapentin in the management of chemotherapy-induced peripheral neuropathy: a phase 3 randomized, double-blind, placebo-controlled, crossover trial (N00C3). Cancer 110(9):2110–2118

50. Wiffen PJ, Derry S, Moore RA et al (2014) Carbamazepine for chronic neuropathic pain and fibromyalgia in adults. Cochrane Database Syst Rev 4:CD005451. doi:10.1002/14651858. CD005451.pub3

51. Barton DL, Wos EJ, Qin R et al (2011) A double blind, placebo-controlled trial of a topical treatment for chemotherapy-induced peripheral neuropathy: NCCTG trial N06CA. Support Care Cancer 19(6):833–841

52. Storey DJ, Colvin LA, Boyle D et al (2011) Topical menthol: a novel intervention that improved chemotherapy induced peripheral neuropathy (CIPN) related pain and physical function. Support Care Cancer 19:S158. (suppl 2; abstr 263)

53. Nakamura M, Onikubo T, Kamikawa H et al (2012) Phase II study of topical menthol for chemotherapy-induced peripheral neuropathy (CIPN). Ann Oncol S9; 23:ix513

54. Stubblefield MD, Burstein HJ, Burton AW (2009) NCCN task force report: management of neuropathy in cancer. J Natl Compr Canc Netw 7(S5):S1–S26

Postradiation Pain Syndromes

55. Mohiuddin JJ, Baker BR, Chen RC (2015) Radiotherapy for high-risk prostate cancer. Nat Rev Urol 12(3):145–154

56. Hennequin C, Guillerm S, Quero L (2015) Radiotherapy in elderly patients, recommendations for the main localizations:

breast, prostate and gynaecological cancers. Cancer Radiother 19(6–7):397–403

57. Marte GR, Cameron N, Kersten C et al (2014) Palliative pelvic radiotherapy of symptomatic incurable rectal cancer — a systematic review. Acta Oncol 53:164–173

58. Willett CG, Ooi CJ, Zietman AL et al (2000) Acute and late toxicity of patients with inflammatory bowel disease undergoing irradiation for abdominal and pelvic neoplasms. Int J Radiat Oncol Biol Phys 46:995–998

59. Greimel ER, Winter R, Kapp KS et al (2009) Quality of life and sexual functioning after cervical cancer treatment: a long-term follow-up study. Psychooncology 18(5):476–482

60. Vistad I, Cvancarova M, Kristensen GB et al (2011) A study of chronic pelvic pain after radiotherapy in survivors of locally advanced cervical cancer. J Cancer Surviv 5(2):208–216

61. O'Connor MJ (2015) Targeting the DNA damage response in cancer. Mol Cell 60(4):547–560

62. Ree AH, Redalen KR (2015) Personalized radiotherapy: concepts, biomarkers and trial design. Br J Radiol 88(1051):20150009

63. Fuccio L, Guido A, Andreyev HJ (2012) Management of intestinal complications in patients with pelvic radiation disease. Clin Gastroenterol Hepatol 10:1326–1334.e4

64. Klee M, Thranov I, Machin PD (2000) The patients' perspective on physical symptoms after radiotherapy for cervical cancer. Gynecol Oncol 76(1):14–23

65. Bye A, Trope C, Loge JH et al (2000) Health-related quality of life and occurrence of intestinal side effects after pelvic radiotherapy — evaluation of long-term effects of diagnosis and treatment. Acta Oncol 39(2):173–180

66. Ferrigno R, Santos A, Martins LC, Weltman E, Chen MJ et al (2010) Comparison of conformal and intensity modulated radiation therapy techniques for treatment of pelvic tumors. Analysis of acute toxicity. Radiat Oncol 5:117

67. Kwon JW, Huh SJ, Yoon YC et al (2008) Pelvic bone complications after radiation therapy of uterine cervical cancer: evaluation with MRI. AJR Am J Roentgenol 191(4):987–994

68. Baxter NN, Habermann EB, Tepper JE (2005) Risk of pelvic fractures in older women following pelvic irradiation. JAMA 294(20):2587–2593

69. Hauer-Jensen M, Denham JW, Andreyev HJN (2014) Radiation enteropathy — pathogenesis, treatment, and prevention. Nat Rev Gastroenterol Hepatol 11(8):470–479

70. Andreyev HJ, Wotherspoon A, Denham JW et al (2010) Defining pelvic-radiation disease for the survivorship era. Lancet Oncol 11:310–312

71. Herold DM, Hanlon AL, Hanks GE (1999) Diabetes mellitus: a predictor for late radiation morbidity. Int J Radiat Oncol Biol Phys 43:475–479

72. Ross JG, Hussey DH, Mayr NA et al (1993) Acute and late reactions to radiation therapy in patients with collagen vascular diseases. Cancer 71:3744–3752

73. Dearnaley DP, Khoo VS, Norman AR et al (1999) Comparison of radiation side-effects of conformal and conventional radiotherapy in prostate cancer: a randomised trial. Lancet 353:267–272

74. Putta S, Andreyev HJ (2005) Faecal incontinence: a late side-effect of pelvic radiotherapy. Clin Oncol (R Coll Radiol) 17:469–477

75. Wallner K, Elliott K, Merrick G (2004) Chronic pelvic pain following prostate brachytherapy: a case report. Brachytherapy 3(3):153–158

76. Bergmark K, Avall-Lundqvist E, Dickman PW et al (2002) Patient-rating of distressful symptoms after treatment for early cervical cancer. Acta Obstet Gynecol Scand 81(5):443–450

77. Klimek M, Kosobucki R, Luczynska E et al (2012) Radiotherapy-induced lumbosacral plexopathy in a patient with cervical cancer: a case report and literature review. Contemp Oncol (Pozn) 16(2):194–196

78. Yi SK, Mak W, Yang CC et al (2012) Development of a standardized method for contouring the lumbosacral plexus: a preliminary dosimetric analysis of this organ at risk among 15 patients treated with intensity-modulated radiotherapy for lower gastrointestinal cancers and the incidence of radiation-induced lumbosacral plexopathy. Int J Radiat Oncol Biol Phys 84(2):376–382

79. Jaeckle KA (2004) Neurological manifestations of neoplastic and radiation-induced plexopathies. Semin Neurol 24(4):385–93

80. Jaeckle KA (2010) Neurologic manifestations of neoplastic and radiation-induced plexopathies. Semin Neurol 30(3):254–262

81. Tsushima T, Nasu Y, Saika T et al (2001) Optimal starting time for flutamide to prevent disease flare in prostate cancer patients treated with gonadotropin-releasing hormone agonist. Urol Int 66:135–139

82. Ackery D, Yardley J (1993) Radionuclide-targeted therapy for the management of metastatic bone pain. Semin Oncol 20:27–31

83. Robinson RG, Preston DF, Spicer JA et al (1992) Radionuclide therapy of intractable bone pain: emphasis on strontium-89. Semin Nucl Med 22:28–32

84. Hird A, Chow E, Zhang L, Wong R et al (2009) Determining the incidence of pain flare following palliative radiotherapy for symptomatic bone metastases: results from three canadian cancer centers. Int J Radiat Oncol Biol Phys 75(1):193–197

85. Loblaw DA, Wu JS, Kirkbride P et al (2007) Pain flare in patients with bone metastases after palliative radiotherapy—a nested randomized control trial. Support Care Cancer 15(4):451–455

86. Gomez-Iturriaga A, Cacicedo J, Navarro A et al (2015) Incidence of pain flare following palliative radiotherapy for symptomatic bone metastases: multicenter prospective observational study. BMC Palliat Care 14:48

87. Hirano Y, Nakamura N, Zenda S et al (2016) Incidence and severity of adverse events associated with re-irradiation for spine or pelvic bone metastases. Int J Clin Oncol 21(3): 609–614

88. Bubley GJ (2001) Is the flare phenomenon clinically significant? Urology 58:5–9

89. Higginson IJ, McCarthy M (1993) Validity of the support team assessment schedule: do staffs' ratings reflect those made by patients or their families? Palliat Med 7:219–228

90. Slevin ML, Plant H, Lynch D et al (1988) Who should measure quality of life, the doctor or the patient? Br J Cancer 57:109–112

91. Chiang A, Zeng L, Zhang L et al (2013) Pain flare is a common adverse event in steroid-naive patients after spine stereotactic body radiation therapy: a prospective clinical trial. Int J Radiat Oncol Biol Phys 86:638–642

92. Hird A, Zhang L, Holt T et al (2009) Dexamethasone for the prophylaxis of radiation-induced pain flare after palliative radiotherapy for symptomatic bone metastases: a phase II study. Clin Oncol (R Coll Radiol) 21(4):329–335

93. Chow E, Meyer RM, Ding K et al (2015) Dexamethasone in the prophylaxis of radiation-induced pain flare after palliative radiotherapy for bone metastases: a double-blind, randomised placebo-controlled, phase 3 trial. Lancet Oncol 16(15): 1463–1472

94. Yousef AA, El-Mashad NM (2014) Pre-emptive value of methylprednisolone intravenous infusion in patients with vertebral metastases. A double-blind randomized study. J Pain Symptom Manage 48(5):762–769

Chronic Postsurgical Pain and Postsurgical Pain Syndromes

95. Kehlet H, Jensen TS, Woolf CJ (2006) Persistent postsurgical pain: risk factors and prevention. Lancet 367(9522):1618–1625

96. Macrae WA (2001) Chronic pain after surgery. Br J Anaesth 87:88–98

97. Macrae WA (2008) Chronic post-surgical pain: 10 years on. Br J Anaesth 101:77–86

98. Andersen KG, Kehlet H (2011) Persistent pain after breast cancer treatment: a critical review of risk factors and strategies for prevention. J Pain 12(7):725–746

99. Hartvigsen J, Christensen K, Frederiksen H (2004) Genetic and environmental contributions to back pain in old age: a study of 2,108 danish twins aged 70 and older. Spine 29:897–901

100. Diatchenko L, Slade GD, Nackley AG et al (2005) Genetic basis for individual variations in pain perception and the development of a chronic pain condition. Hum Mol Genet 14:135–143

101. Zubieta JK, Heitzeg MM, Smith YR et al (2003) COMT val-158met genotype affects mu-opioid neurotransmitter responses to a painstressor. Science 299:1240–1243

102. Mogil JS, Wilson SG, Chesler EJ et al (2003) The melanocortin-1 receptor gene mediates female-specifi c mechanisms of analgesia in mice and humans. Proc Natl Acad Sci U S A 100(8):4867–4872

103. Yang Z, Yang Z, Arheart KL et al (2012) CYP2D6 poor metabolizer genotype and smoking predict severe postoperative pain in female patients on arrival to the recovery room. Pain Med 13(4):604–609

104. Devor M, Raber P (1990) Heritability of symptoms in an experimental model of neuropathic pain. Pain 42:51–67

105. Young EE, Lariviere WR, Belfer I (2012) Genetic basis of pain variability: recent advances. J Med Genet 49(1):1–9

106. Sorge RE, Trang T, Dorfman R et al (2012) Genetically determined P2X7 receptor pore formation regulates variability in chronic pain sensitivity. Nat Med 18(4):595–599

107. Nissenbaum J, Devor M, Seltzer Z et al (2010) Susceptibility to chronic pain following nerve injury is genetically affected by CACNG2. Genome Res 20(9):1180–1190

108. Costigan M, Belfer I, Griffin RS et al (2010) Multiple chronic pain states are associated with a common amino acid-changing allele in KCNS1. Brain 133(9):2519–2527

109. Turk DC, Okifuji A (1996) Perception of traumatic onset, compensation status, and physical findings: impact on pain severity, emotional distress, and disability in chronic pain patients. J Behav Med 19:435–453

110. Linton SJ, Overmeer T, Janson M et al (2002) Graded in vivo exposure treatment for fear-avoidant pain patients with functional disability: a case study. Cogn Behav Ther 31:49–58

111. Hanley MA, Jensen MP, Ehde DM et al (2004) Psychosocial predictors of long-term adjustment to lower-limb amputation and phantom limb pain. Disabil Rehabil 26:882–893

112. Granot M, Ferber SG (2005) The roles of pain catastrophizing and anxiety in the prediction of postoperative pain intensity: a prospective study. Clin J Pain 21:439–445

113. Katz J, Poleshuck EL, Andrus CL et al (2005) Risk factors for acute pain and its persistence following breast cancer surgery. Pain 119:16–25

114. Okifuji A, Donaldson G, Barck L et al (2010) Relationship between fibromyalgia and obesity in pain, function, mood, and sleep. J Pain 11:1329–1337

115. Omoigui S (2007) The biochemical origin of pain—proposing a new law of pain: the origin of all pain is inflammation and the inflammatory response—a unifying law of pain. Med Hypotheses 69:70–82

116. Joshi I, Ogunnaike BO (2005) Consequences of inadequate pain relief and chronic persistent postoperative pain. Anesthesiol Clin North America 23:21–36

117. Gehling M, Scheidt CE, Niebergall H et al (1999) Persistent pain after elective trauma surgery. Acute Pain 2:110–114

118. Campbell CM, France CR, Robinson ME et al (2008) Ethnic differences in diffuse noxious inhibitory controls. J Pain 9:759–766

119. Edwards RR, Ness TJ, Weigent DA (2003) Individual differences in diffuse noxious inhibitory controls (DNIC): Association with clinical variables. Pain 106:427–437

120. Perkins FM, Kelhet H (2000) Chronic pain as an outcome from surgery. A review of predictive factors. Anesthesiology 93:1123–1133

121. Katz J, Seltzer Z (2009) Transition from acute to chronic post-surgical pain: risk factors and protective factors. Expert Rev Neurother 9:723–744

122. Peters ML, Sommer M, de Rijke JM et al (2007) Somatic and psychologic predictors of long-term unfavorable outcome after surgical intervention. Ann Surg 245:487–494

123. Buvanendran A, Kroin JS, Kerns JM et al (2004) Characterization of a new animal model for evaluation of persistent post-thoracotomy pain. Anesth Analg 99:1453–1460

124. Brandsborg B (2012) Pain following hysterectomy: epidemiological and clinical aspects. Dan Med J 59(1):B4374

125. Macrae WA, Davies HTO (1999) Chronic postsurgical pain. In: Crombie IK, Linton S, Croft P (eds) Epidemiology of pain. IASP Press, Seattle, WA, pp 125–142

126. Merskey H, Bogduk H et al (1994) Classification of chronic pain: descriptions of chronic pain syndromes and definitions of pain terms. IASP Press, Seattle, WA

127. Woolf CJ, Ma Q (2007) Nociceptors-noxious stimulus detectors. Neuron 55:353–364

128. Bhave G, Gereau RW (2004) Posttranslational mechanisms of peripheral sensitization. J Neurobiol 61:88–106

129. Ji RR, Kohno T, Moore KA et al (2003) Central sensitization and LTP: do pain and memory share similar mechanisms. Trends Neurosci 26:696–705

130. D'Mello R, Dickenson AH (2008) Spinal cord mechanisms of pain. Br J Anaesth 101:8–16

131. Aasvang E, Kehlet H (2005) Chronic postoperative pain: the case of inguinal herniorrhaphy. Br J Anaesth 95:69–76

132. Jung BF, Ahrendt GM, Oaklander AL et al (2003) Neuropathic pain following breast cancer surgery: proposed classification and research update. Pain 104:1–13

133. Liu CN, Raber P, Ziv-Sefer S et al (2001) Hyperexcitability in sensory neurons of rats selected for high versus low neuropathic pain phenotype. Neuroscience 105:265–275

134. Messelink B, Benson T, Berghmans B et al (2005) Standardization of terminology of pelvic floor muscle function and dysfunction: report from the pelvic floor clinical assessment group of the International Continence Society. Neurourol Urodyn 24(4):374–380

135. Vodusek DB (2004) Anatomy and neurocontrol of the pelvic floor. Digestion 69(2):87–92

136. Andromanakos NP, Kouraklis G, Alkiviadis K (2011) Chronic perineal pain: current pathophysiological aspects, diagnostic approached and treatment. Eur J Gastroenterol Hepatol 23(1):2–7

137. Prendergast SA, Weiss JM (2003) Screening for musculoskeletal causes of pelvic pain. Clin Obstet Gynecol 46(4):773–782

138. Weiss JM (2000) Chronic pelvic pain and myofascial trigger points. Pain Clin 2(6):13–18

139. Ovesen P, Krøner K, Ornsholt J et al (1991) Phantom-related phenomena after rectal amputation: prevalence and clinical characteristics. Pain 44(3):289–291

140. Fingren J, Lindholm E, Carlsson E (2013) Perceptions of phantom rectum syndrome and health-related quality of life in patients following abdominoperineal resection for rectal cancer. J Wound Ostomy Continence Nurs 40(3):280–286

141. Rashiq S, Dick BD (2014) Post-surgical pain syndromes: a review for the non-pain specialist. Can J Anaesth 61(2):123–130

142. Grant AM, Scott NW, O'Dwyer PJ (2004) MRC Laparoscopic Groin Hernia Trial Group. Five-year follow-up of a randomized trial to assess pain and numbness after laparoscopic or open repair of groin hernia. Br J Surg 91(12):1570–1574

143. Tsunoda AT, Andrade CE, Vieira MA et al (2015) Laparoscopy in uterine cervical cancer. Current state and literature review. Rev Col Bras Cir 42(5):345–351

144. Nezhat FR, Pejovic T, Finger TN (2013) Role of minimally invasive surgery in ovarian cancer. J Minim Invasive Gynecol 20(6):754–765

145. Scheib SA, Fader AN (2015) Gynecologic robotic laparoendoscopic single-site surgery: prospective analysis of feasibility, safety, and technique Am J Obstet Gynecol 212(2):179.e1–8. doi: 10.1016/j.ajog.2014.07.057

146. Clarke H, Bonin RP, Orser BA et al (2012) The prevention of chronic postsurgical pain using gabapentin and pregabalin: a combined systematic review and meta-analysis. Anesth Analg 115(2):428–442

147. Chaparro LE, Smith SA, Moore RA (2013) Pharmacotherapy for the prevention of chronic pain after surgery in adults. Cochrane Database Syst Rev 7:CD008307.doi:10.1002/14651858. CD008307.pub2

148. Sen H, Sizlan A, Yanarates O et al (2009) A comparison of gabapentin and ketamine in acute and chronic pain after hysterectomy. Anesth Analg 109(5):1645–1650

149. Sen H, Sizlan A, Yanarates O et al (2009) The effects of gabapentin on acute and chronic pain after inguinal herniorrhaphy. Eur J Anaesthesiol 26(9):772–776
150. Singla NK, Chelly JE, Lionberger D et al (2014) Pregabalin for the treatment of postoperative pain: results from three controlled trials using different surgical models. J Pain Res 8:9–20
151. Woolf CJ, Chong MS (1993) Preemptive analgesia—treating postoperative pain by preventing the establishment of central sensitization. Anesth Analg 77(2):362–379
152. Kissin I, Bright CA, Bradley EL Jr (2000) The effect of ketamine on opioid-induced acute tolerance: can it explain reduction of opioid consumption with ketamine-opioid analgesic combinations? Anesth Analg 91(6):1483–1488
153. Katz J, Schmid R, Snijdelaar DG et al (2004) Pre-emptive analgesia using intravenous fentanyl plus low-dose ketamine for radical prostatectomy under general anesthesia does not produce short-term or long-term reductions in pain or analgesic use. Pain 110(3):707–718
154. Fassoulaki A, Sarantopoulos C, Melemeni A et al (2001) Regional block and mexiletine: the effect on pain after cancer breast surgery. Reg Anesth Pain Med 26(3):223–228
155. Katz J, Cohen L (2004) Preventive analgesia is associated with reduced pain disability 3 weeks but not 6 months after major gynecologic surgery by laparotomy. Anesthesiology 101(1):169–174
156. Fassoulaki A, Triga A, Melemeni A (2005) Multimodal analgesia with gabapentin and local anesthetics prevents acute and chronic pain after breast surgery for cancer. Anesth Analg 101(5):1427–1432
157. Lavand'homme P, De Kock M, Waterloos H (2005) Intraoperative epidural analgesia combined with ketamine provides effective preventive analgesia in patients undergoing major digestive surgery. Anesthesiology 103(4):813–820
158. Anderson RU, Harvey RH, Wise D et al (2015) Chronic pelvic pain syndrome: reduction of medication use after pelvic floor physical therapy with an internal myofascial trigger point wand. Appl Psychophysiol Biofeedback 40(1):45–52

Chapter 4
Pain Assessment

While pain is a highly subjective experience, its management necessitates objective standards of care. Consequently, patient's painful experience assessment is a crucial moment during pain management and makes it efficient [1]. Patient assessment refers to the complete history and features of the painful experience achieved through questions about location, duration (constant or intermittent), onset, radiation, associated symptoms, severity, quality (e.g., sharp pains, cramping, dull aching pain), and alleviating and aggravating factors [2]. In the latter case, a key step in pain assessment is the evaluation of the effectiveness of pharmacologic and non-pharmacologic therapy. Moreover, we must investigate on other factors, like movement, bowel movements, physical therapy, activity, sexual activity, mental anguish, depression, sadness, that may cause or intensify the pain.

The physical examination should include a thorough neurological examination, while the psychosocial assessment is important to discriminate pain in the context of other non-pain symptoms (e.g., anxiety, mood, sleep, cancer-related fatigue) and suffering [3].

A special issue in the pain management concerns the pain assessment tools used to elicit responses by patients about their comfort or discomfort, to enhance the clarity in communications, and to support an individualized pain management program. For this purpose, physicians can use a wide range of tools, divided into unidimensional and multidimensional scales [4].

© Springer International Publishing Switzerland 2016   63
M. Cascella et al., *Features and Management of the Pelvic Cancer Pain*, DOI 10.1007/978-3-319-33587-2_4

Unidimensional scales fill this role by providing fast (often one item) measures of pain; they can be administered multiple times with minimal administrative effort. The most commonly used unidimensional tool is the NRS. Although variations exist, the instrument typically consists of scores from 0 to 10 (or 0–100), with the far left being described as "no pain" and the far right described as "worst pain imaginable." The NRS has the advantage of being administered verbally, thus not requiring patient mobility. VAS is an easy-to-use psychometric response scale alternative to the NRS. The patient marks anywhere along a 10-cm line to indicate their current pain intensity, which can be measured in millimeters to yield a 101-point scale. To assist in the scoring process, slide rule-like device has been developed. VRS is another tool for pain assessment; it is sometimes used for individuals who have trouble translating their pain experience into a number value. The scores are replaced with descriptors, such as no pain, mild pain, moderate pain, and severe pain.

In many situations, a simple, one-item instrument is not sufficient to define either pain or the link between pain intensity and disability. For this purpose, multidimensional instruments are more suitable as well as more comprehensive than rating scales [5]. These tools measure several dimensions of pain, with differing combinations of pain intensity, quality, affect, interference with functioning, and effects on general QoL. The McGill Pain Questionnaire [6] and especially the short-form McGill Pain Questionnaire [7] are validated measures for pain assessment used widely. Both are self-report questionnaires which can be used to monitor the pain over time and to determine the effectiveness of any intervention. The questionnaire consists primarily of three major classes of word descriptors (sensory, affective, and evaluative) used by patients to specify subjective pain experience. It also contains an intensity scale and other items to determine the properties of pain experience.

Additionally, other tools have been developed. The BPI was designed by the Pain Research Group of the WHO Collaborating Centre for Symptom Evaluation in Cancer

Care [8]. It captures the sensory intensity of pain and the QoL pain related with 15 total descriptors concerning presence (1 item), sites (1 item) and severity of pain (4 items), status (1 item) and effects of pain treatment (1 item), and interference of pain in QOL (7 items). The Pain Management Index (PMI) is a measure of the appropriateness of pharmacological strategies and compares the potency of prescribed analgesic medications using patient-reported pain levels. Analgesics are classified into four levels: 0: no analgesic; 1: nonopioid; 2: weak opioid; 3: strong opioid. Pain levels are scored as follows: 1–3: mild; 4–7: moderate; and 8–10: severe. PMI scores are calculated by subtracting patient-reported pain levels from analgesic levels, which produces a score range of −3 to 3. Negative scores (<0) indicate inadequate analgesia and positive scores (≥0) indicate adequate analgesia [9].

Other multidimensional instruments used for assessment of cancer pain in specific clinic conditions are the German pain questionnaire for children and adolescents (DSF-KJ), the West Haven-Yale Multidimensional Pain Inventory (WHYMPI) with 52 items and 12 subscales [10] used for, for example, dysfunctional and depressed patients, the 120 items Treatment Outcomes of Pain Survey (TOPS) more suitable for patients with chronic pain [11], and the Alberta Breakthrough Pain Assessment Tool specifically designed for BTcP in the clinical trial setting [12].

Among the symptom assessment tools developed to correlate pain with depression, fatigue, and other symptoms commonly seen in those with cancer, we cite the Distress "Thermometer," which is a modified visual analog scale designed to look like a thermometer, with 0 meaning "no distress" and 10 (at the top of the thermometer) indicating "extreme distress." Accompanying the thermometer scale is a checklist, including a variety of physical, psychological, practical, family support, and spiritual/religious concerns [13] (Fig. 4.1).

Other pain assessment tools are the behavioral pain scales, often used in noncommunicative patients, such as deeply sedated and mechanically ventilated patients in intensive

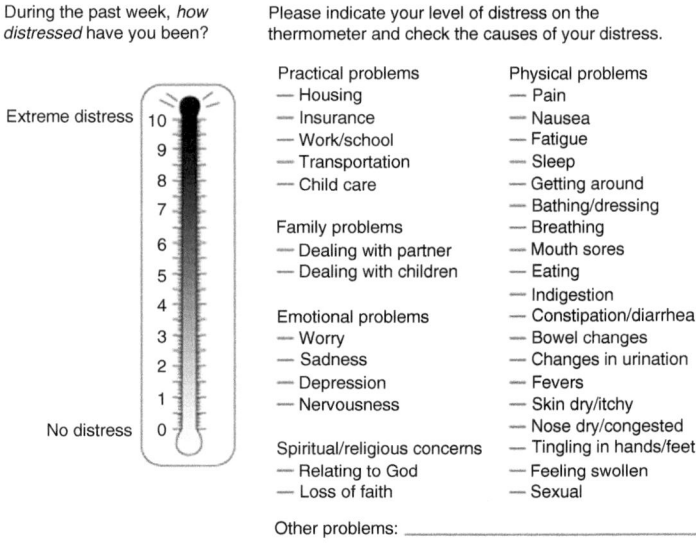

During the past week, *how distressed* have you been?

Please indicate your level of distress on the thermometer and check the causes of your distress.

Extreme distress — 10
9
8
7
6
5
4
3
2
1
No distress — 0

Practical problems
— Housing
— Insurance
— Work/school
— Transportation
— Child care

Family problems
— Dealing with partner
— Dealing with children

Emotional problems
— Worry
— Sadness
— Depression
— Nervousness

Spiritual/religious concerns
— Relating to God
— Loss of faith

Physical problems
— Pain
— Nausea
— Fatigue
— Sleep
— Getting around
— Bathing/dressing
— Breathing
— Mouth sores
— Eating
— Indigestion
— Constipation/diarrhea
— Bowel changes
— Changes in urination
— Fevers
— Skin dry/itchy
— Nose dry/congested
— Tingling in hands/feet
— Feeling swollen
— Sexual

Other problems: _____

FIGURE 4.1. Distress "thermometer"

care unit (ICU) to assess the sedation and the analgesia [14], or in young children to assess the postoperative pain [15]. These tools measure facial and bodily movements as proxies for pain in association with other clinical measurements, such as the compliance to mechanical ventilation in ICU patients, or the crying and the consolability in children.

According to Herr and colleagues [16], every effort should be made to elicit self-reporting of cancer pain. A study revealed that 22 % of patients said that their healthcare professionals never, or only occasionally, asked them about their pain [17]. Thus, every effort to elicit self-reporting of pain must be made. If a patient is unable to comply with pain assessment tools or to explain his/her pain verbally, other stratagems can be used, for instance, asking the patient to blink once to indicate if pain is present and twice if not [18].

Especially in patients in palliative care setting, pain assessment should be associated with assessment of physical function. For this purpose, the Karnofsky performance status scale and the Oncology Group scale are less effective than other tools, such as the Edmonton Functional Assessment tool [19] and the Palliative Performance Scale (PPS) [20]. The Edmonton tool includes domains such as pain, mental alertness, communication, sensory function, and respiratory function. Moreover, this tool could be particularly effective in patients affected by cancer diseases of the pelvis because it explores also the patient's mobility. PPS is substantially a modification of the Karnofsky scale which provides domains useful for pelvic patient assessment, including ambulation and activity.

Unfortunately, there is not a specific examination, tool, or quantifiable methods measuring patient's pain level objectively; the patient's pain experience assessment often is the integration of several data obtained by observational behavior, physiological findings, and patient self-reporting information.

Because an accurate pain assessment is the first major step necessary for good cancer pain management [21], and failure to assess pain is a critical factor leading to undertreatment [22], the characteristics of pain assessment have been summarized in a dedicated table (Table 4.1).

TABLE 4.1. Pain history[a]

Location(s)
Onset
Duration (constant or intermittent)
Radiation
Associated symptoms
Severity (unidimensional and multidimensional tools)
Quality (aching, throbbing, squeezing, cramping, burning, tingling, etc.)
Alleviating factors (pharmacologic and non-pharmacologic therapy, position, etc.)
Aggravating factors (movement, physical therapy, activity, mental anguish, depression, sadness, etc.)
Temporal Pattern
Continuous
Intermittent Pain
• Incident (associated with a known precipitating event or BTcP)
• Non-incident (spontaneous or BTcP)
End-of-dose failure (occurs just before a scheduled opioid dose)

(continued)

TABLE 4.1. (continued)

ᵃRecommendations for pain assessment:

1. Combine pain history with *neurological examination* (e.g., altered sensation) and *psychosocial assessment* (cultural factors, existential distress, etc.)
2. Use one or more pain assessment tools (also multidimensional)
3. Make every effort to elicit self-reporting of pain
4. Assess cancer pain, response to the therapy, and QoL at the same time. For example, large doses of opioids may be needed to eliminate pain in some patients, but this approach can induce considerable levels of side effects
5. If possible, try to distinguish the components of the pain, as this can help you in the choice of therapy [*strong recommendation for management of pelvic cancer pain*]
6. Record every change in pain history
7. Record medication history
8. Especially in patients in palliative care setting assess also the physical function

References

1. McCracken K (2015) The challenges of cancer pain assessment. Ulster Med J 84(1):55–57
2. Fink R (2000) Pain assessment: the cornerstone to optimal pain management. Proc (Bayl Univ Med Cent) 13(3):236–239
3. Breivik H, Borchgrevink PC, Allen SM et al (2008) Assessment of pain. Br J Anaesth 101(1):17–24
4. Younger J, McCue R, Mackey S (2009) Pain outcomes: a brief review of instruments and techniques. Curr Pain Headache Rep 13(1):39–43
5. Scottish Intercollegiate Guidelines Network (2008) Control of pain in adults with cancer: a national clinical guideline. Guideline 106. http://www.sign.ac.uk/pdf/SIGN106.pdf. Accessed Sept 2015
6. Melzack R (1975) The McGill Pain Questionnaire: major properties and scoring methods. Pain 1(3):277–299
7. Melzack R (1987) The short-form McGill Pain Questionnaire. Pain 30:191–197

8. Cleeland CS, Ryan KM (1994) Pain assessment: global use of the Brief Pain Inventory. Ann Acad Med Singapore 19:129–138

9. Charles S, Cleeland RG, Alan KH et al (1994) Pain and its treatment in outpatients with metastatic cancer. N Engl J Med 330:592–596

10. Kerns RD, Turk DC, Rudy TE (1985) The West Haven-Yale Multidimensional Pain Inventory (WHYMPI). Pain 23:345–356

11. Rogers WH, Wittink H, Wagner A et al (2000) Assessing individual outcomes during outpatient multidisciplinary chronic pain treatment by means of an augmented SF-36. Pain Med 1:44–54

12. Hagen NA, Stiles C, Nekolaichuk C et al (2008) The Alberta Breakthrough Pain Assessment Tool for cancer patients: a validation study using a delphi process and patient think-aloud interviews. J Pain Symptom Manage 35(2):136–152

13. O'Donnell E (2013) The distress thermometer: a rapid and effective tool for the oncology social worker. Int J Health Care Qual Assur 26(4):353–359

14. Payen JF, Bru O, Bosson JL (2001) Assessing pain in critically ill sedated patients by using a behavioral pain scale. Crit Care Med 29(12):2258–2263

15. Merkel SI, Voepel-Lewis T, Shayevitz JR et al (1997) The FLACC: a behavioral scale for scoring postoperative pain in young children. Pediatr Nurs 23(3):293–297

16. Herr K, Coyne PJ, Key T et al (2006) Pain assessment in the nonverbal patient: position statement with clinical practice recommendations. Pain Manag Nurs 7(2):44–52

17. Breivik H, Cherny N, Collett B et al (2009) Cancer-related pain: a pan-European survey of prevalence, treatment, and patient attitudes. Ann Oncol 20(8):1420–1433

18. Merkel S (2002) Pain assessment in infants and young children: the finger span scale. Am J Nurs 102(11):55–56

19. Kaasa T, Loomis J, Gillis K et al (1997) The Edmonton Functional Assessment Tool: preliminary development and evaluation for use in palliative care. J Pain Symptom Manage 13(1):10–19

20. Anderson F, Downing GM, Hill J et al (1996) Palliative Performance Scale (PPS): a new tool. J Palliat Care 12(1):5–11, Spring

21. Bruera E, Kim HN (2003) Cancer pain. JAMA 290(18):2476–2479

22. Herr K, Titler MG, Schilling ML et al (2004) Evidence based assessment of acute pain in older adults: current nursing practices and perceived barriers. Clin J Pain 20(5):331–340

Part II
Treatments

Chapter 5
Pharmacological Approaches

Guidelines have been developed to assist providers in assessing and treating the cancer pain [1, 2]. Analgesics, particularly opioids, are the mainstay of cancer pain treatment, but it is possible to use a great variety of drugs, such as NSAIDs, acetaminophen, and several adjuvant drugs. In 1986, the World Health Organization (WHO) established a three-step ladder as a guideline for the treatment of cancer pain [3]. The document was translated into 22 different languages and has served as an incentive for increasing the awareness in the world about the importance of pain treatment in cancer patients [4]. It was demonstrated that this ladder provides an adequate analgesia in 90 % of cancer patients [5] and in more than 75 % of terminally ill cancer patients [6]. It proposes a stepwise optimization of systemic pharmacotherapy which uses NSAIDs or acetaminophen at the first, followed by opioid agents. More precisely, this guideline provides recommendations for analgesic selection (non-opioid, weak opioid, and strong opioid) based on level of pain (mild, moderate, and severe). Tests of the analgesic ladder suggest that the compliance of the guidelines with a multimodal pharmacological approach is significant [7, 8]. In any case, despite the availability of these guidelines, cancer pain continues to be managed in many patients inadequately [9].

© Springer International Publishing Switzerland 2016
M. Cascella et al., *Features and Management of the Pelvic Cancer Pain*, DOI 10.1007/978-3-319-33587-2_5

According to WHO guideline, the first step of the pain therapy refers to "mild to moderate pain" with the use of non-opioid drugs, like NSAIDs or acetaminophen. NSAIDs have anti-inflammatory, analgesic, and antipyretic effects, acting on the arachidonic and eicosapentaenoic acid metabolism which are the precursors of prostaglandins, prostacyclin, thromboxanes, and leukotriene involved in inflammation. Moreover, these drugs potentiate the beta-endorphin action and antagonize the substance P effect. Acetaminophen stops, as NSAIDs, prostaglandin's synthesis but it does not act on the peripheral inflammation site, but only on CNS.

While non-opioid drugs alone usually do not provide sufficient relief for patients with pelvic cancer pain, a better result is obtained by associating them with adjuvant drugs, medication with a primary indication different from pain, but with some analgesic properties in some painful conditions. These medicaments (e.g., tricyclic antidepressants, benzodiazepines, corticosteroids, anticonvulsants) usually are coadministered with other analgesics in each step of pain management and they are particularly helpful in specific clinical conditions, such as patients with neuropathic pain.

Antidepressants are considered drugs of choice for the treatment of lancinating but also dull neuropathic pain especially, because of its continuing burning component. The analgesic effects of antidepressants may be determined by different events: the inhibition of the serotonin and norepinephrine CNS reuptake resulting in the activation of pain modulation descending pathways, the sodium channels block in the site where the ectopic discharges originate, and the improvement of opioid binding to specific receptors that reduces the tolerance phenomenon [10].

The results of a Cochrane review on nortriptyline do not support the use of this drug as a first-line treatment for neuropathic pain [11], despite duloxetine [12] and pregabalin [13] achieved a better result. The outcome of at least 50 % pain intensity reduction was regarded as a useful outcome of treatment by patients, and the achievement of this degree of pain relief was associated with important beneficial effects on sleep interference, fatigue, and depression, as well as QoL, function, and work. The antiepileptic action mechanism is not completely understood yet, but the analgesic effect on neuropathic pain seems to depend on different mechanisms: the sodium channels and NMDA receptors block, the inhibition of voltage activated-calcium channels, the increase of the inhibitory activity through the interaction with GABA-A receptors, the inhibition of presynaptic glutamate release, and the suppression of spontaneous ectopic neuronal discharges [14].

Commonly, corticosteroids are used for the treatment of the pain due to peripheral nerve injury or nerve/plexus infiltration and compression, because of the prostaglandin's synthesis inhibition and decreasing firing from injured nerves. With this action, the pain signals diminish from periphery to spinal cord or from spinal cord to brain. Steroids also decrease capillary permeability, thereby reducing edema and the mass effect of the lesion. In pelvic diseases, they are often added to enhance analgesia for pain from bone metastasis.

Many patients with advanced pelvic cancer have "moderate to severe chronic pain" (step 2). In this case, the WHO analgesic ladder for cancer pain management advises the use of weak opioids (e.g., codeine) with or without non-opioids. Codeine is an opiate used for its analgesic, antitussive, antidiarrheal, anxiolytic, antidepressant, sedative, and hypnotic properties. Because codeine acts only after cytochrome P450 enzyme CYP2D6 metabolism to morphine, patients either who lack this enzyme or who are taking drug inhibitors of its function will get no pain relief. Medications capable of reducing, or even completely blocking, the codeine to morphine conversion are two selective serotonin reuptake inhibitors, paroxetine, and fluoxetine, as well as the antihistamine diphenhydramine and the antidepressant bupropion. Many of these drugs are administered in cancer patient frequently.

Tramadol is a weak opioid with selective binding for the μ-opioid receptors about 10-fold lower than codeine and 6000-fold lower than morphine [15]. Nevertheless, a non-opioid mechanism is also involved in tramadol analgesia, consisting of the enhancement of the descending monoaminergic systems involved in the inhibition of pain. This action is achieved through interference with the noradrenalin and serotonin uptake and their extra neural concentration increase. Codeine and tramadol can be adequate drugs for the management of mild cancer and non-cancer pain; however, cancer pain (especially pelvic cancer pain) is rarely mild to be controlled using these drugs.

Although codeine and tramadol are drugs adopted widely, in this step it is possible to utilize strong opioids, such as oxycodone with or without naloxone; however, these drugs should be administered at the lowest effective dose.

Cancer pelvic pain is a "severe pain" almost always, identifying the third step of the WHO analgesic ladder in which the use of strong opioids is recommended.

The term opioid indicates, in pharmacology, a family of synthetic substances able to modify the emotional response and the perception pain due to their ability to bind specific receptors of the nervous system defined opioid receptors. Morphine is the founder, and it is the reference point in the evaluation of analgesic activity of its other congeners. The opioids analgesic effect is the result of several mechanisms, such as the direct inhibition of ascending transmission of nociceptive information from the spinal cord dorsal horn, the activation of the control pain circuits stemming from the midbrain to the dorsal horn of the spinal cord, the action in the brain (limbic system), and the affective modulation of pain perception [16].

Examples of step 3 opioids are oxycodone, morphine, fentanyl, methadone, tapentadol, and hydromorphone. Management of opioids foresees the expertise of the provider who must evaluate type of drug, dose, route(s) of administration, side effects, and specific pharmacokinetic phenomena, such as the opioid-induced dependence and tolerance.

Pain management is obtained case-by-case and with a dynamic assessment. The provider plays associating, circling, and changing different medications with different durations of action. The so-called "around the clock" opioid therapy, which is defined as medication that is given at regularly scheduled intervals throughout the day (in contrast to medication that is given only as needed, see Sect. 6.1 Breakthrough cancer pain management) is recommended by all the recent guidelines, such as those of the European Society of Clinical Oncology (ESMO) [17] and the European Association for Palliative Care (EAPC) [18], as first-line therapy in patients with cancer in order to achieve sufficient pain control.

Oxycodone has similar efficacy to morphine and according to ESMO and EAPC guidelines, modified-release oxycodone formulations for oral administration are an effective first-choice alternative to oral morphine in patients with moderate to severe cancer pain.

Like other opioids, the primary disadvantage associated with oxycodone is the development of bowel dysfunction in many patients, which commonly manifests as significant constipation [19]. Treatment guidelines strongly recommend routine laxative use for both the prophylaxis and the management of opioid-induced constipation in patients with advanced cancer receiving opioid therapy. In patients who are unresponsive to laxatives, opioid antagonists such as methylnaltrexone are used as second-line agents to prevent and treat opioid-induced gastrointestinal effects. Methylnaltrexone bromide antagonizes the opioids' action on the gastrointestinal tract. It has limited ability to cross the blood brain barrier; therefore, this drug has a selective peripheral action on μ-opioid receptors in the gastrointestinal tract without interfering with opioid-mediated analgesic effects on the central nervous system [20].

A first method to antagonize the opioids effects on peripheral receptors was the use of immediate release naloxone, given orally or parenterally. The results were, however, unsatisfactory because constipation improved but the naloxone was rapidly absorbed and it reached the CNS in sufficient quantity to interfere with the analgesic effect and to determine abstinence's crisis [21]. According to our previous investigations, a fixed-dose combination opioid agonist/antagonist therapy (oxycodone/naloxone) could preserve bowel function in patients with chronic cancer pain, without the CNS absorption [22].

Peripheral opioid antagonists offer two distinct advantages for the prevention of opioid side effects. First, they do not reverse centrally mediated analgesia, and secondly, a single drug could be used to prevent multiple adverse side effects. They represent a target therapy, intending as a therapy based on the removal of the constipation's causes which, in the case of the induced opioid constipation, are iatrogenic. The laxative therapy, however, is only a symptomatic therapy; it does not act on the cause of the problem. Therefore, these drugs represent a sure advance in medical therapy.

The EAPC working group identified four general approaches to consider when encountering adverse effects caused by opioids: dose reduction of systemic opioid, symptomatic management of the adverse effect, opioid rotation, and switching the route of systemic administration [23]. All opioids are associated with several adverse effects, but the incidence and severity vary from opioid to opioid. Tolerance to some of these adverse effects can develop (e.g., nausea/vomiting), but not to others, like constipation. The latter complication affects 95 % of patients treated with morphine and 50 % with fentanyl. It is inevitable and persistent; thus, a laxative should be prescribed prophylactically *starting at the same time as the opioid*. On the other hand, nausea/vomiting are less frequent (30–50 % of morphine patients). They usually manifest themselves in the first 5–10 days until tolerance develops. Also drowsiness (20 % of patients) usually persists for the first 3–5 days until tolerance develops.

Side effects of opioids and their ameliorations are shown in Table 5.1, while Table 5.2 offers some suggestions for opioid equivalents.

TABLE 5.1 Side effects of opioids and amelioration

Common side effects	Amelioration
Ileus/constipation	Stool softeners (Docusate sodium) [a]Laxatives (osmotic, saline, stimulant) Use opioid antagonists or a fixed-dose combination opioid agonist/antagonist therapy Switch the way the opioid is given (e.g., transdermal fentanyl)
Dry mouth	Mouth care: frequent sips of iced drinks, dental floss, saliva replacements, or stimulants
Nausea/vomiting	Antiemetic (serotonin antagonists; Haloperidol 0.5–1.5 mg at night; Cyclizine 25–50 mg three times daily) Prokinetic agents ([b]Metoclopramide 10 mg three times daily)
Sedation (with initiation of opioid therapy or with dose increases)	Decrease the dose of the opioid, switch to a different opioid, or switch the way the opioid is given

Less common Side effects	Amelioration
Edema and sweating	Switch opioids
Respiratory depression	Decrease the dose of the opioid, switch to a different opioid, or switch the way the opioid is given
Urinary retention	Titrate dose Switch opioids
Cough suppression	Titrate dose Switch opioids
Dizziness	Antivertiginous agents
Confusion/delirium/ hallucinations	Titrate dose Switch opioids Antipsychotics (Haloperidol, Chlorpromazine)

(continued)

TABLE 5.1 (continued)

Less common Side effects	Amelioration
Tolerance/dependence	Switch opioids [Long-acting preparations (transdermal fentanyl) and possibly some forms of other slow release opioids]
Pruritus	Switch opioids Antihistamines Paroxetine
Endocrine dysfunction/ reduced libido	Switch opioids Endocrine monitoring

[a]The dose of laxative should be titrated to maintain the patient's normal pattern of bowel opening
[b]Avoid metoclopramide in case of bowel obstruction

TABLE 5.2 Opioids equivalents[a]

Codeine	60 mg oral = 6 mg oral morphine
Tramadol	100 mg oral = 10 mg oral morphine
Oxycodone	5 mg oral = 10 mg oral morphine 4 mg sc = 5 mg sc morphine
Hydromorphone	7.5 mg oral = 1.5 mg parenteral
Fentanyl	50–100 mg oral morphine/die = 25 mcg/h transdermal fentanyl 25 mcg/h iv fentanyl = 25 mcg/h transdermal fentanyl (1:1)

Equianalgesic morphine parenteral:oral = 1:2 or 1:3

Equianalgesic oxycodone parenteral:oral = 1:2

Equianalgesic hydromorphone parenteral:oral = 1:2

[a]In table, "single doses" equivalences, i.e., only equivalents in single-dosed healthy volunteers, are reported. Equivalent in chronically dosed sick patients is difficult to quantify

Some Practical Suggestions

Start Low and Go Slow. Opioids should be started at low doses and titrated up gradually to reach the point of maximum pain relief with minimum side effects.
In older patients, the starting dose is usually lowered.
Starting dose and Titration:

- Start with oral normal-release morphine 2.5–5 mg every 4 h (15–30 mg/die) in opioid naïve, elderly, and cachectic patients, *or*
- with oral normal-release morphine 5 mg every 4 h (30 mg/die) in patients using a WHO step II opioid.
- Titration: increase 25–50–100 %/24 h (the incremental percentage decreases as the dose increases), but consider the side effects.
- During the morphine titration phase, use pain assessment tools
- Keep a record of the amount taken, and once a stable dosing regimen is achieved (generally 2–3 days) convert to a long-acting preparation by calculating the total 24-h dose of immediate release required, divide by two, and give twice daily.
- Remember:
  - Opioid naïve patient refers to an individual who has either never had an opioid or who has not received repeated opioid dosing for a 2–3 week period.
  - Oral opioid titration and intravenous opioid titration are equally effective.
  - There is no upper dose for morphine use unless the patient suffers from distressing and uncontrollable side effects.
  - *Normal-release* morphine is the same of *immediate-release* referred to in some texts.
  - Hydrate the patient to avoid morphine toxicity.

Warning! Opioid Medications to Avoid In Older Adults

- *Meperidine*: a metobolite produces CNS toxicity that may cause tremor, irritability, cognitive changes, and seizures.
- *Propoxyphene*: long half-life, metabolite causes CNS and cardiac toxicity and can cause renal injury.
- *Pentazocine*: causes delirium and agitation in older patients, potential for renal injury.

5.1   Breakthrough Cancer Pain Management

Opioids used for the management of BTcP should provide a rapid onset of analgesic action and duration, appropriate for the characteristics of the BTcP episodes. Moreover, due to its nature, BTcP requires a treatment that is appropriate in its potency and is easily administered. As interindividual variability is an important factor, the ideal treatment should cover every BTcP episode.

BTcP is often managed by oral morphine in doses of about 1/6 of the daily opioid regimen. For instance, morphine sulfate oral liquid formulation shows an onset time of 15–30 min and reaches its peak effect in 1 h. Nevertheless, newer technologies have been developed to provide a rapid onset of effect with potent opioid drugs, such as fentanyl, delivered through sublingual, buccal, and intranasal routes of administration.

Fentanyl is a potent opioid analgesic approximately 100 times more potent than morphine, and its strong potency, in relation to that of morphine, is largely due to its high lipophilicity. It is a strong agonist at the μ-opioid receptors and has a rapid onset and short duration of action. In this approach, the use of the so-called rapid onset opioids (ROOs), also called transmucosal immediate-release fentanyl drugs, is increasingly widespread. Moreover, a recent randomized, crossover, controlled study showed that the use of ROO (fentanyl buccal tablet) in doses proportional to the opioid regimen for background pain was clearly superior for efficacy and rapidity in comparison with oral morphine [24], and other authors demonstrated that administration of sublingual fentanyl might provide a more effective treatment option than oral morphine [25].

Several delivery systems are available today, and many more are under development. They use different routes of administration, but none of them is oral. Compared to the oral route, these preparations offer a big advantage: because the drug is absorbed directly into the systemic circulation, the first-pass effect is avoided.

ROOs can be grouped into two broad categories based on the route of administration: buccal/sublingual and nasal. Among the different ROOs, intranasal fentanyl shows a quicker onset to analgesia than buccal tablets, which in turn has a quicker onset to analgesia than oral transmucos alfentanyl citrate [26]. Intranasal fentanyl has also a higher bio-availability (60–89 %) compared to sublingual (70 %) and buccal (50–60 %).

Determining the exact dosage of opioid (also ROO) in BTcP management is a paramount problem, given the choice between dose titration and proportional doses to the basal opioid regimen. About ROOs, although some authors suggested that the dose should be individually titrated to enable effective analgesia [27], proportional doses seem to be more effective and safer, especially in patients receiving higher doses of opioids for background pain [28]. Thus, according to Mercadente et al. [24, 29], a dose of 100 µg of fentanyl buccal tablet (or oral morphine 10 mg, as alternative to ROO) can be delivered to patients receiving 60 mg of oral morphine as basal opioid regimen, 200 µg of ROO (or 20 mg of oral morphine) in patients receiving 120 mg of basal oral morphine, 300 µg ROO (or 30 mg of oral morphine) in patients receiving 180 mg of basal oral morphine, and so on.

The non-oral routes of opioid administration include also rectal and parenteral (intravenous, subcutaneous) modalities. Although oral/sublingual and intranasal routes are the favorite methods of administrations for the BTcP, intravenous morphine is the quickest route to control BTcP and in some clinical conditions has been found to be highly effective and safe [30]. Nevertheless, this approach is feasible in palliative acute units, but in most other centers is not favorite and at home injections are not easily manageable. Subcutaneous route is commonly preferred in a hospice setting, although the onset of action may be not fast enough. Hydromorphone has been delivered subcutaneously using a "pain pen" [31].

Practical Suggestions for BTcP Management

- Control background pain (with around the clock analgesia).
- Optimal management of BTcP requires independent assessment and targeted treatment.
- Combining long-acting opioids, used to control background analgesia, with ROOs seem to be the most appropriate choice for BTcP management.
- In case of oral morphine, or ROOs, use proportional doses to basal opioid regimen.
- Intravenous morphine is the quickest route to control BTcP and in some clinical conditions has been found to be highly effective and safe.

5.2   Pharmacological Approaches for Bone Metastasis

This is a significant issue, as pain caused by cancer within bones is one of the most serious forms of pain, and most of the painful pelvic cancer syndromes are caused by bone metastasis, from breast, kidney, prostate, thyroid or lung, or by multiple myeloma. Other than pain, bone metastases cause significant complications, including pathological fracture, spinal cord compression, nerve root compression, and hypercalcemia, so treatments for painful osseous metastases may not only diminish pain but also may improve QoL.

Multidisciplinary approaches are usually adopted in the palliation of bone metastases. Accordingly, the appropriate treatment strategy is the result of a thorough assessment and the application of a pharmacological, radiotherapeutic, orthopedic, or minimally invasive approaches is evaluated after a case-by-case analysis.

Pharmacological approaches include opioids, anticonvulsants (gabapentin and pregabalin), topiramate, bisphosphonates (BPs), monoclonal antibodies (denosumab), and hormonal therapy (for breast and prostate cancers).

The rationale of the use of anticonvulsants is the evidence that peripheral nerve destruction can take place in bone, and the growth of metastatic lesions in bone appears to lead to a complex sensory nerve injury characterized by sprouting of sensory fibers into bone, upregulation of galanin and glial fibrillary acidic protein with hypertrophy of satellite cells surrounding ipsilateral DRG sensory neuron cell bodies, and ipsilateral DRG macrophage infiltration [32].

Topiramate is an antiepileptic drug which is particularly well suited for the treatment of painful osseous metastases, since in addition to its multiple mechanisms of action, it also possesses actions as a carbonic anhydrase inhibitor. Topiramate is a calcium channel blocker, sodium channel blocker, glutamic acid inhibitor, and GABA facilitator and may affect the NMDA receptor complex. Adequate hydration is recommended due to the potential formulation of calcium phosphate renal stones.

BPs, like zoledronic acid, pamidronate, and ibandronate, are pyrophosphate analogues with anti-proliferative, anti-angiogenic, and apoptotic properties [33]. These drugs bind avidly to the hydroxyapatite bone mineral surfaces and are internalized selectively by osteoclasts [34], thereby altering the cytoskeleton and inducing loss of actin rings that lead to osteoclast apoptosis. According to the Second Cambridge Conference on metastatic bone cancer, BPs reduce cancer bone pain in 50 % of recipients regardless of the primary tumor [35] and should be considered where analgesics and/or radiotherapy are inadequate for the management of painful bone metastases [36]. Among the BPs, zoledronic acid is the only drug that has statistically shown significant reductions in skeletal morbidity, including bone pain, in patients with metastatic prostate cancer [37]. Zoledronic acid can cause flu-like symptoms that are manageable with standard treatment, and it may be used with caution in patients with impaired renal function. Osteonecrosis of the jaw is a serious adverse effect.

Denosumab is a human monoclonal IgG2 antibody that binds to receptor activator of nuclear factor kappa-B ligand (RANKL) with high affinity and specificity; this plays a central role in the mediation of bone resorption and remodeling RANKL. Denosumab is used to prevent fracture, spinal cord compression, or to reduce the bone's radiation or surgery need in patients with bone solid tumors metastases from, but with multiple myeloma metastases. In patients with advanced breast cancer and bone metastases, denosumab showed improvement in pain prevention and comparable pain palliation compared with BPs. In addition, fewer denosumab-treated patients shifted to strong opioid analgesic therapy [38]. Hypocalcemia is a problem connected with the denosumab administration because this drug can significantly reduce the blood calcium levels, in fact, some deaths have been reported [39]. In literature, there is also a report of rhabdomyolysis followed by acute kidney injury after acute exposure to denosumab and abiraterone [40], the latter commonly used as an adrenal androgen synthesis inhibitor in cancer prostate.

Hormone therapy is a therapeutic approach for hormone-sensitive prostate cancer; indeed, it can relieve pain, prevent pathologic fractures, and prevent neurologic complications from bone metastases. Androgen deprivation therapy is achievable with surgical castration (bilateral orchiectomy) or medical castration through drugs such as synthetic gonadotropin releasing hormone (GrRH) agonists (e.g., leuprolide, buserelin, and triptorelin), androgen receptor antagonists (e.g., bicalutamide, nilutamide, flutamide), or inhibitors of 5α-reduction (e.g., finasteride, dustasterude). Side effects of hormone treatments depend on the type of treatment used. The most common side effect for many of these treatments is hot flashes. Hormone treatment for prostate cancer can lead to anemia, weight gain, and loss of sex drive.

Potential future therapeutic agents are Cannabinoid Receptor-2 (CBR2) agonists, such as JWH015, because they have been shown to act as an analgesic in acute, chronic, and neuropathic pain [41]. Additionally, CB2 agonists have been shown to increase bone density by increasing the number of osteoblasts and, at the same time, by inhibiting the production of osteoclasts [32, 42].

5.3   The Fourth Step of the WHO Ladder

Is the WHO therapeutic guideline for pain management still a valid tool? For most patients with cancer pain, the WHO three-step analgesic ladder provides adequate management with oral or transdermal options. However, some cancer patients are not well pain controlled with these approaches, and several problems have been identified with use of the ladder. As an instance, in the treatment of bone pain, many pain specialists believe that the second step is useless and a progress should rapidly be made toward the third step, as patient condition dictates [43].

Perhaps, the most important deficiency in the ladder is that it does not address those patients who have failed oral or transdermal options. In 1996, WHO proposed an update which provided a better explanation of the pathophysiology of pain, focusing on the assessments of pain, the choice of the analgesics, and the use of the ladder [44].

Since then, several proposed modifications of the WHO diagram have been made. Eisenberg et al. [45] suggested the elimination of the second level. Other authors recommend modifications and adaptations of the analgesic scale for other

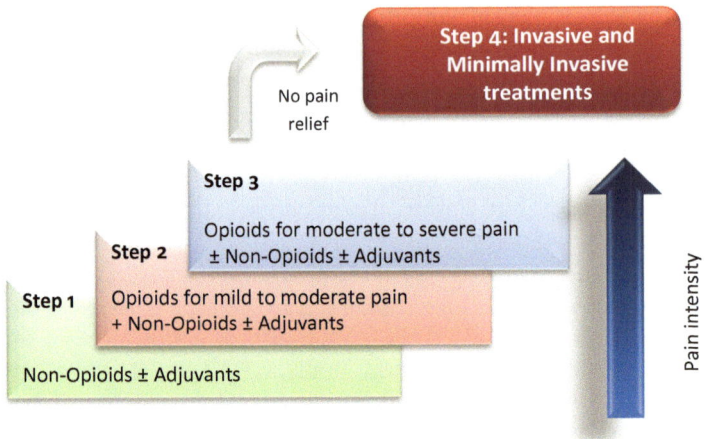

FIGURE 5.1 Modified WHO analgesic ladder

types of pain, such as acute pain and chronic non-cancer pain [46, 47]. About the QoL, some authors have devised an innovative revision with the integration of a fourth step [48]. This fourth step is an "interventional" step and includes invasive techniques, for example, spinal (epidural and subarachnoid) administration of local anesthetics, nerve blocks, and neurolysis (e.g., phenolization, alcoholization, thermocoagulation, and radiofrequency) or neurosurgical procedures, such as spinal cord stimulation [49] (Fig. 5.1). This adapted model has also been proposed and applied in the treatment of pediatric pain [50].

The issue concerning the interventional step for pain management is of paramount importance in pelvic neoplasms. For instance, in patients affected by pelvic bone metastasis, it is mandatory to obtain pain relief with the best possible QoL despite the advanced stage of disease. This target must be achieved especially in case of osteolytic lesions in the periacetabular region, as they can provoke pathological fractures and subsequent functional impairment [51]. For this purpose, if the patient is eligible for surgery, one of the several reconstruction techniques for the pelvis can be applied, depending on the

TABLE 5.3 Recommendations for pharmacologic pain management

Consider comorbidities[a]
Pay attention to the side effects
Follow the WHO analgesic ladder, but consider that in pelvic cancer pain most palliative care patients require stronger analgesics at the beginning
Choose the easier route of administration
Control background pain following the *around the clock* opioid therapy
Switch opioids
Switching route can sometimes help[b]
Use adjuvants
Manage breakthrough cancer pain, as it is a serious problem for the patient
Consider bisphosphonates and monoclonal antibodies for bone metastasis
Consider opioid equivalents (see Table 5.2)
Personalize treatment

[a]In renally impaired patients, start with lower-than-recommended doses of opioids and slowly titrate up the dose while extending the dosing interval

[b]Remember in case of switch to fentanyl patch, the original opioid should be continued for 12 h as fentanyl takes effect

patient's prognosis size of the bone defect in order to restore the mechanical stability of the hip joint and preserve the mobility [51] (see also Appendix B. Algorithm for Pelvic Cancer Pain Management).

General recommendations for pharmacologic pain management are shown in Table 5.3.

References

1. Jacox A, Carr DB, Payne R et al (1994) Management of cancer pain. Clinical practice guideline. No 9. AHCPR Publication No 94-0592. Rockville
2. Miaskowski C, Cleary J, Burney R et al (2005) Guideline for the management of cancer pain in adults and children. APS clinical practice guideline series, No 3. American Pain Society, Glenview

3. World Health Organization (1986) Cancer pain relief. WHO Publications Center, Geneva

4. Miller E (2004) The World Health Organization analgesic ladder. J Midwifery Womens Health 49(6):542–545

5. Ventafridda V, Caraceni A, Gamba A (1990) Field-testing of the WHO guidelines for cancer pain relief: summary report of demonstration projects. Adv Pain Res Ther 16:451–464

6. Grond S, Zech D, Schug SA, Lynch J et al (1991) Validation or World Health Organization guidelines for cancer pain relief during the last days and hours of life. J Pain Symptom Manage 6:411–422

7. Jadad AR, Browman GP (1995) The WHO analgesic ladder for cancer pain management. Stepping up the quality of its evaluation. JAMA 274(23):1870–1873

8. Zech DF, Grond S, Lynch J et al (1995) Validation of World Health Organization guidelines for cancer pain relief: a 10-year prospective study. Pain 63:65–76

9. Cleeland CS, Mendoza TR, Wang XS et al (2000) Assessing symptom distress in cancer patients: the M.D. Anderson Symptom Inventory. Cancer 89:1634–1646

10. Saarto T, Wiffen PJ (2007) Antidepressants for neuropathic pain. Cochrane Database Syst Rev 4:CD005454. doi:10.1002/14651858. CD005454.pub2

11. Derry S, Wiffen PJ, Aldington D et al (2015) Nortriptyline for neuropathic pain in adults. Cochrane Database Syst Rev 1:CD011209. doi:10.1002/14651858.CD011209.pub2

12. Lunn MP, Hughes RA, Wiffen PJ (2014) Duloxetine for treating painful neuropathy, chronic pain or fibromyalgia. Cochrane Database Syst Rev 1:CD007115. doi:10.1002/14651858. CD007115.pub3

13. Moore RA, Wiffen PJ, Derry S et al (2014) Gabapentin for chronic neuropathic pain and fibromyalgia in adults. Cochrane Database Syst Rev 4:CD007938. doi:10.1002/14651858. CD007938.pub3

14. Inturrisi CE (2002) Clinical pharmacology of opioids for pain. Clin J Pain 18(Suppl 4):S3–S13

15. Elliott JA (2010) Opioids in the management of acute pain. In: Elliott JA, Smith HS (eds) Handbook of acute pain management. Taylor & Francis, Boca Raton, FL, p 84

16. Eisenberg E, River Y, Shifrin A et al (2007) Antiepileptic drugs in the treatment of neuropathic pain. Drugs 67(9): 1265–1289

17. Ripamonti CI, Santini D, Maranzano E et al (2012) Management of cancer pain: ESMO clinical practice guidelines. Ann Oncol 23(Suppl 7):vii139–vii154

18. Caraceni A, Hanks G, Kaasa S, European Palliative Care Research Collaborative (EPCRC), European Association for Palliative Care (EAPC) (2012) Use of opioid analgesics in the treatment of cancer pain: evidence-based recommendations from the EAPC. Lancet Oncol 13(2):e58–e68

19. Camilleri M (2011) Opioid-induced constipation: challenges and therapeutic opportunities. Am J Gastroenterol 106(5):835–843

20. Thomas J, Karver S, Cooney GA et al (2008) Methylnaltrexone for opioid-induced constipation in advanced illness. N Engl J Med 358:2332–2343

21. Sykes NP (1996) An investigation of the ability of oral naloxone to correct opioid-related constipation in patients with advanced cancer. Palliat Med 10(2):135–144

22. Cuomo A, Russo G, Esposito G et al (2014) Efficacy and gastrointestinal tolerability of oral oxycodone/naloxone combination for chronic pain in outpatients with cancer: an observational study. Am J Hosp Palliat Care 31(8):867–876

23. Cherny N, Ripamonti C, Pereira J et al (2001) Strategies to manage the adverse effects of oral morphine: an evidence-based report. J Clin Oncol 19:2542–2554

24. Mercadante S, Adile C, Cuomo A et al (2015) Fentanyl buccal tablet vs. oral morphine in doses proportional to the basal opioid regimen for the management of breakthrough cancer pain: a randomized, crossover, comparison study. J Pain Symptom Manage 50(5):579–586

25. Velázquez Rivera I, Muñoz Garrido JC, García Velasco P (2014) Efficacy of sublingual fentanyl vs. oral morphine for cancer-related breakthrough pain. Adv Ther 31(1):107–117

26. Jandhyala R, Fullarton JR, Bennett MI (2013) Efficacy of rapid-onset oral fentanyl formulations vs. oral morphine for cancer-related breakthrough pain: a meta-analysis of comparative trials. J Pain Symptom Manage 46(4):573–580

27. Davies A, Dickman A, Reid C (2009) The management of cancer-related breakthrough pain: recommendations of a task group of the Association of Palliative Medicine of Great Britain and Ireland. Eur J Pain 13:331–338

28. Mercadante S, Gatti A, Porzio G et al (2012) Dosing fentanyl buccal tablet for breakthrough cancer pain: dose titration versus proportional doses. Curr Med Res Opin 28:963–968

29. Mercadante S, Villari P, Ferrera P et al (2007) Transmucosal fentanyl vs. intravenous morphine in doses proportional to basal opioid regimen for episodic-breakthrough pain. Br J Cancer 96:1828–1833

30. Mercadante S, Intravaia G, Villari P et al (2008) Intravenous morphine for episodic-breakthrough pain in an acute palliative care unit: a confirmatory study. J Pain Symptom Manage 35:307–313

31. Enting RH, Mucchiano C, Oldenmenger WH et al (2005) The "pain pen" for breakthrough cancer pain: a promising treatment. J Pain Symptom Manage 29:213–217

32. Smith HS (2012) Painful boney metastases. Ann Palliat Med 1(1):14–31

33. Clezardin P (2011) Bisphosphonates' antitumor activity: an unravelled side of a multifaceted drug class. Bone 48:71–79

34. Russell RG, Rogers MJ, Frith JC et al (1999) The pharmacology of bisphosphonates and new insights into their mechanisms of action. J Bone Miner Res 14:53–65

35. Coleman RE, Guise TA, Lipton A et al (2008) Advancing treatment for metastatic bone cancer: consensus recommendations from the Second Cambridge Conference. Clin Cancer Res 14:6387–6395

36. Wong R, Wiffen PJ (2002) Bisphosphonates for the relief of pain secondary to bone metastases. Cochrane Database Syst Rev 2:CD002068. doi:10.1002/14651858.CD002068

37. Furlow B (2006) Zoledronic acid palliation in bone-metastatic breast cancer. Lancet Oncol 7:894

38. Sun L, Yu S (2013) Efficacy and safety of denosumab versus zoledronic acid in patients with bone metastases: a systematic review and meta-analysis. Am J Clin Oncol 36(4):399–403

39. Peddi P, Lopez-Olivo MA, Pratt GF (2013) Denosumab in patients with cancer and skeletal metastases: a systematic review and meta-analysis. Cancer Treat Rev 39(1):97–104

40. Neyra JA, Rocha NA, Bhargava R et al (2015) Rhabdomyolysis-induced acute kidney injury in a cancer patient exposed to denosumab and abiraterone: a case report. BMC Nephrol 16:118. doi:10.1186/s12882-015-0113-6

41. Whiteside GT, Lee GP, Valenzano KJ (2007) The role of the cannabinoid CB2 receptor in pain transmission and therapeutic potential of small molecule CB2 receptor agonists. Curr Med Chem 14:917–936

42. Ofek O, Karsak M, Leclerc N et al (2006) Peripheral cannabinoid receptor, CB2, regulates bone mass. Proc Natl Acad Sci U S A 103:696–701

43. Miguel R (2000) Interventional treatment of cancer pain: the fourth step in the World Health Organization analgesic ladder? Cancer Control 7(2):149–156

44. World Health Organization (1996) Cancer pain relief with a guide to opioid availability. WHO Publications Center, Geneva

45. Eisenberg E, Marinangeli F, Birkhahm J et al (2005) Time to modify the WHO analgesic leader? Pain Clin Update 13(5):1–4

46. Gómez-Cortéz MD, Rodríguez-Huertas F (2000) Reevaluación del segundo escalón de la escalera analgésica de la OMS. Rev Soc Esp Dolor 7(6):343–344

47. Vargas-Schaffer G (1999) Manejo y tratamiento del doloroncológico. In: Vargas-Schaffer G, Esposito Quercia G (eds) Dolor y cuidados paliativos en oncologia. evaluación, manejo y tratamiento. EdicionesExpansiónCientífica G&S, Caracas, pp 79–93

48. Vargas-Schaffer G (2010) Is the WHO analgesic ladder still valid? Twenty-four years of experience. Can Fam Physician 56(6):514–517

49. Christo PJ, Mazloomdoost D (2008) Interventional pain treatments for cancer pain. Ann N Y Acad Sci 1138:299–328

50. Krakowski I, Falcoff H, Gestin Y et al (1996) Recommandation pour une bonne pratique dans la prise en charge de la douleur du cancer chez l'adulte et l'enfant. Bull Cancer 83(Suppl 1):1S–84S

51. Müller DA, Capanna R (2015) The surgical treatment of pelvic bone metastases. Adv Orthop 2015:525363. doi:10.1155/2015/525363

Chapter 6
Palliative Radiotherapy

RT can provide safe, cost-effective, efficient palliation of various symptoms of advanced cancer with minimal side effects, also in pelvic cancer diseases. Approximately, one-half of the RT prescribed in the USA is delivered with palliative intent; among these patients, 40 % suffered from cancer prostate and 12 % had a colorectal cancer [1].

Because there are several approaches for palliative RT, the choice depends on a case-by-case analysis, through the evaluation of the tumor site, biological and histological features of the disease, prognosis, performance status, eventual comorbidities, psychological issues, and availability of resources. Furthermore, location and symptomatic site are indexed to the relative effectiveness of each palliative RT intervention. Indeed, not always the responses are optimal because pain caused by visceral or lymph-vascular involvement (or both) responds more rapidly than the more refractory neuropathic pain due to plexus (e.g., sacral plexus) involvement [2].

Although old studies suggested that two-dimensional (2D) external beam radiotherapy (EBRT) with a dose of 45 Gy could improve pain with low toxicity risk to the small intestine [3], however, this radiotherapic approach exposes larger amounts of tissue, including normal tissues, to high doses of radiation.

Over the last 30 years, radiotherapy has undergone great technological progress going from 2D-EBRT to three-dimensional CRT, IMRT, and stereotactic radiotherapy (SBRT)/radiosurgery (SRS).

© Springer International Publishing Switzerland 2016   95
M. Cascella et al., *Features and Management of the Pelvic Cancer Pain*, DOI 10.1007/978-3-319-33587-2_6

The 3D-CRT utilizes cross-sectional imaging to develop a plan maximizing dose to the target volume while minimizing dose to surrounding tissue. Indeed, the majority of patients will get clinical benefit from two-dimensional or three-dimensional conformal EBRT with moderate doses of radiation, like 8 Gy in a single fraction to 30 Gy in 10 fractions or 35–37.5 Gy in 14–15 fractions [4]. These treatments are often associated with minimal side effects. Probably, it is possible to reduce the dose; in fact, Valeriani and colleagues showed a high rate of pain relief with lower incidence of acute toxicity in patients affected by painful bone metastases of spine, sacrum, or pelvis who were treated with 20 Gy in 5 fractions compared with those treated through 30 Gy in 10 fractions [5].

The IMRT uses a computer algorithm to create multiple small beams to generate highly conformal plans. It optimizes the delivery of irradiation to irregularly shaped volumes and has the ability to produce concavities in radiation treatment volumes. This advanced approach of RT can be delivered using linear accelerators (LINAC) with static multileaf collimators (step and shoot IMRT), dynamic multileaf collimators, volumetric modulated arc therapy (VMAT), or tomotherapy machines. Although prostate cancer is one of the most common tumor sites treated with IMRT worldwide [6], IMRT has been evaluated in other pelvic malignancies including anal and rectal cancer, as well as cervix and endometrial cancers [7], and muscle-invasive carcinoma of the bladder, in the latter also with palliative intent [8]. Moreover, IMRT techniques could play a role for pain palliation of chemotherapy-resistant ovarian cancer [9] and for treating some types of painful pelvic cancer bone, such as Ewing's sarcoma [10].

The SBRT/SRS is a new technique that allows to deliver high doses to the target with concurrent sparing of the surrounding normal tissue in a few fractions using a coordinate system. SBRT/SRS can be performed with a LINAC dedicated with a Gamma Knife (for intracranial lesions) and with

Cyberknife® System (for intracranial and extracranial lesions). In pelvis, the role of SBRT, for instance, in reirradiation of pelvic recurrences of rectal cancer, is yet poorly investigated. It seems to improve local control and palliate local symptoms with limited normal tissue toxicity and short treatment time [11]. Nevertheless, while these new advanced approaches can potentially improve symptom control and durability, they are associated with increased technical and economic costs.

Although in locally advanced and recurrent rectal cancers pain relief is the major indication for palliative pelvic EBRT, studies report a general underutilization of palliative RT for this purpose [12]. Moreover, currently there is no consensus on how palliative EBRT of rectal cancer should optimally be delivered in terms of optimal dose and fractionation. As a general principle, treatments can be given both as single fractions and more commonly fractionated over several weeks (up to 9 weeks). The most commonly used fraction dose is 2 Gy (range 1.5–10 Gy) and total doses range from 5 to 70 Gy, most often in the range of 30–60 Gy [13]. Symptomatic responses were reported at low total doses of radiotherapy ($\leq$20 Gy) during the course of fractionated treatment and after single fractions of 5–10 Gy. Several authors reported no difference in palliative effect across a range of radiotherapy prescriptions [13].

Radiation therapy is quite effective in giving relief from the painful bone metastasis in patients with multiple osteoblastic lesions and osteolytic or mixed lesions in ilium and pubis. Studies reported that 50–80 % of patients experience improvement in their pain, and 20–50 % of the treated patients have even complete pain relief [14]. For these evidences, the external irradiation should be the standard care for patients with localized bone pain, resulting in the palliation of the majority of these patients. Anyway, some patients do not experience any pain relief. Furthermore, patients who have recurrent pain at a site previously irradiated may not be eligible for further radiation therapy by reason of the limitation in normal tissue tolerance. About the palliative RT modality, a systematic review showed no significant differences between single fractions and multiple fractions in terms of response rates and no significant differences with respect to acute toxicities were observed. However, a significantly higher re-treatment rate with single fractions was evident [15].

A prospective multicenter study on symptomatic incurable prostate cancer showed that in the majority of patients, palliative pelvic RT with 30–39 Gy contributes to relief pain and improves QoL with acceptable toxicity [16].

Brachytherapy, also known as internal radiotherapy, sealed source radiotherapy, curietherapy, or endocurietherapy, is a form of RT where a sealed radiation source is placed inside or next to the area requiring treatment to deliver temporary or permanent highly conformal radiation. In pelvic cancers, brachytherapy is commonly used as an effective treatment for cervical and prostate cancers; nevertheless, it can also be used in local tumor control and symptom palliation to treat locally recurrent anorectal tumors [17].

Internal therapy by bone seeking radiopharmaceuticals, such as Rhenium (Re)-1861 or Radium-223, is one of the optional treatments for palliation of painful bone metastases in patients with multifocal bone lesions which cannot be treated by EBRT [18]. Nevertheless, these treatments can lead to several side effects, like reversible myelosuppression, which may be significant, and the treatments should not be given to patients with suspected disseminated intravascular coagulation.

All these clinical evidences showed that palliative external or internal RT is one of the most effective methods for symptomatic control in advanced cancer patients. Nevertheless, as demonstrated by a survey among the members of the National Hospice and Palliative Care Organization and American Society for Therapeutic Radiology and Oncology, multiple barriers, like RT, transportation difficulties, short life expectancy, and educational deficiencies between the specialties limit the use of palliative RT in hospice care; thus, only 10 % of hospice providers consider radiation oncologists to be part of the palliative care team [19]. Another barrier is the fear of side effects by RT. The pain manager must consider both general side effects of RT and the possible side effects occurring during/after RT to the pelvic area (see Sect. 3.2 for postradiation pain syndromes). The former include weakness, fatigue, nausea, fever, and infection, the latter consisting of gastrointestinal (diarrhea, rectal bleeding), genitourinary (radiation cystitis, incontinence), and those affecting skin (skin burns, skin dryness) or connective tissue. Other symptoms, such as impotence in men, changes in menstruation, such as stopping menstruating and vaginal itching, burning and dryness in women are also possible.

As stated in Sect. 3.2, a transient progression of pain, the so-called pain flare, can occur after palliative RT in the treatment of painful bone metastases in approximately 40 % of patients [20]. This painful complication is defined as a two-point increase of the worst pain score on an 11-point rating scale, compared to baseline, without a decrease in analgesic intake, or a 25 % increase in analgesic intake without a decrease in worst pain score [21]. A pain flare is distinguished from progression of pain by requiring the worst pain score and analgesic intake to return to baseline levels after the flare [22]. A recent randomized placebo-controlled, phase 3 trial showed that two 4 mg dexamethasone tablets taken orally at least 1 h before the start of radiation treatment are able to prevent this complication [23].

In case of RT, for locally advanced and recurrent rectal cancers' pain relief, side effects, such as small bowel obstruction, enteritis, or anuria, could be serious; however, data reported regarding old studies performed by supervoltage X-ray therapy [24], while modern radiotherapy planning systems and standardized palliative dose radiotherapy regimens should suggest the limited side effects of these techniques. Moreover, many of the symptoms resolve themselves within a few days or weeks after treatment has finished.

Key Points

- Radiation therapy is quite effective in giving relief from the painful bone metastasis, with a pain response rate of more than 60 %.
- In locally advanced and recurrent rectal cancers, pain relief is the major indication for palliative pelvic EBRT.
- Pain caused by visceral or lymph-vascular involvement (or both) responds more rapidly than the more refractory neuropathic pain due to nerves or plexi (e.g., sacral plexus) involvement.

Practical Suggestions

- After palliative RT, assess the quality of the approach by considering effectiveness on pain in terms of complete, partial, or nonresponse. The latter as stable pain or pain progression.
- Consider the effectiveness of the RT also in terms of reduction of analgesic consumption.
- Be ready to prevent pain flare and manage side effects of RT and their upgrading in combination with those of pharmacologic therapy.

References

1. Murphy JD, Nelson LM, Chang DT et al (2013) Patterns of care in palliative radiotherapy: a population-based study. J Oncol Pract 9(5):e220–e227. doi:10.1200/JOP.2012.000835
2. Ahluwalia A, Janjan NA, Muir C (2010) Radiotherapy and chemotherapy in cancer pain management. In: Fishman SM, Ballantyne JC, Rathmell JP (eds) Bonica's management of pain, 4th edn. Lippincott Williams and Wilkins, Philadelphia, PA, p 646

3. Pacini P, Cionini L, Pirtoli L et al (1986) Symptomatic recurrences of carcinoma of the rectum and sigmoid. The influence of radiotherapy on the quality of life. Dis Colon Rectum 29(12): 865–868

4. Jones JA, Simone CB 2nd (2014) Palliative radiotherapy for advanced malignancies in a changing oncologic landscape: guiding principles and practice implementation. Ann Palliat Med 3(3):192–202. doi:10.3978/j.issn.2224-5820.2014.07.06

5. Valeriani M, Scaringi C, Blasi L et al (2015) Multifraction radiotherapy for palliation of painful bone metastases: 20 Gy versus 30 Gy. Tumori 101(3):318–322

6. Tsai CL, Wu JK, Chao HL et al (2011) Treatment and dosimetric advantages between VMAT, IMRT, and helical tomotherapy in prostate cancer. Med Dosim 36(3):264–271

7. Teoh M, Clark CH, Wood K et al (2011) Volumetric modulated arc therapy: a review of current literature and clinical use in practice. Br J Radiol 84(1007):967–996

8. Whalley D, Caine H, McCloud P et al (2015) Promising results with image guided intensity modulated radiotherapy for muscle invasive bladder cancer. Radiat Oncol 10:205. doi:10.1186/s13014-015-0499-0

9. De Meerleer G, Vandecasteele K, Ost P et al (2011) Whole abdominopelvic radiotherapy using intensity-modulated arc therapy in the palliative treatment of chemotherapy-resistant ovarian cancer with bulky peritoneal disease: a single-institution experience. Int J Radiat Oncol Biol Phys 79(3):775–781

10. Treece SJ, Mukesh M, Rimmer YL et al (2013) The value of image-guided intensity-modulated radiotherapy in challenging clinical settings. Br J Radiol 86(1021):20120278

11. Borzillo V, Falivene S, Di Franco R et al (2016) Role of radiotherapys. In: Romano GM (ed) Multimodal treatment of recurrent pelvic colorectal cancer. Springer, Heidelberg, pp 49–53

12. Jacob S, Wong K, Delaney GP (2010) Estimation of an optimal utilisation rate for palliative radiotherapy in newly diagnosed cancer patients. Clin Oncol (R Coll Radiol) 22(1):56–64

13. Cameron MG, Kersten C, Vistad I (2014) Palliative pelvic radiotherapy of symptomatic incurable rectal cancer—a systematic review. Acta Oncol 53(2):164–173

14. Bates T (1992) A review of local radiotherapy in the treatment of bone metastases and cord compression. Int J Radiat Oncol Biol Phys 23(1):217–221

15. Chow E, Harris K, Fan G et al (2007) Palliative radiotherapy trials for bone metastases: a systematic review. J Clin Oncol 25(11):1423–1436
16. Cameron MG, Kersten C, Vistad I et al (2015) Palliative pelvic radiotherapy for symptomatic incurable prostate cancer—a prospective multicenter study. Radiother Oncol 115(3):314–320
17. Grond S, Zech D, Diefenbach C et al (1996) Assessment of cancer pain: a prospective evaluation of 2266 cancer patients referred to a pain service. Pain 64:107–114
18. Lin Y (2015) Internal radiation therapy: a neglected aspect of nuclear medicine in the molecular era. J Biomed Res 29(5): 345–355
19. Lutz S, Spence C, Chow E et al (2004) Survey on use of palliative radiotherapy in hospice care. J Clin Oncol 22(17):3581–3586
20. Loblaw DA, Wu JS, Kirkbride P et al (2007) Pain flare in patients with bone metastases after palliative radiotherapy—a nested randomized control trial. Support Care Cancer 15(4):451–455
21. Hird A, Chow E, Zhang L et al (2009) Determining the incidence of pain flare following palliative radiotherapy for symptomatic bone metastases: results from three Canadian cancer centers. Int J Radiat Oncol Biol Phys 75(1):193–197
22. Chow E, Ling A, Davis L et al (2005) Pain flare following external beam radiotherapy and meaningful change in pain scores in the treatment of bone metastases. Radiother Oncol 75(1):64–69
23. Chow E, Meyer RM, Ding K et al (2015) Dexamethasone in the prophylaxis of radiation-induced pain flare after palliative radiotherapy for bone metastases: a double-blind, randomised placebo-controlled, phase 3 trial. Lancet Oncol 16(15): 1463–1472
24. Williams IG, Shulman IM, Todd IP (1957) The treatment of recurrent carcinoma of the rectum by supervoltage X-ray therapy. Br J Surg 44:506–508

Chapter 7
Central Neuraxial Blocks

About 85 and 90 % of patients with advanced cancer can have their pain well controlled with the use of analgesic drugs and adjuvants, which usually can be taken orally [1]. However, failure in controlling the symptoms with standard pharmacological pain management requires that multimodal management and invasive techniques should be employed [2]. Several interventions are commonly used for the pelvic or perineal cancer pain treatment, including epidural medications, intrathecal administration of analgesic and local anesthetic drugs through pain pumps, superior and inferior hypogastric plexus blocks, and neurolysis of the Ganglion Impar. In other chapters, we will discuss the features and role of minimally invasive palliative procedures (MIPPs) and neurolytic sympathetic plexus blocks in management of pelvic cancer pain.

Drugs delivery can be achieved with a percutaneous epidural or intrathecal catheter; the latter through an external syringe pump or an implantable intrathecal drug delivery system.

7.1 Epidural Blockade

Epidural blockade is the most practical and widely used continuous method of neural blockade in surgical and obstetric anesthesia. It is the best invasive technique for the management of chronic thoracic, abdominal, and pelvic cancer pain

© Springer International Publishing Switzerland 2016   103
M. Cascella et al., *Features and Management of the Pelvic Cancer Pain*, DOI 10.1007/978-3-319-33587-2_7

thanks to the possibility of drugs administration which selectively block pain conduction, even if leaving sensation and motor function. Several studies showed that epidural analgesia can provide satisfactory pain relief in intractable cancer pain with efficacy varying from 76 to 100 % [3, 4]. Intractable severe pain despite the aggressive pharmacological interventions by conventional administration routes (oral, rectal, transdermal, subcutaneous, and intravenous) or dose-limiting side effects experienced from conventional administration routes is the principal indication to epidural blockade for pain management in cancer patients.

Morphine is the most used drug for epidural way because of its low lipid solubility, slow onset of action, and long duration of analgesia. This opioid is usually administered through a continuous infusion pump principally or through intermittent bolus. In various researches, the addition of a local anesthetic, such as bupivacaine [5] and ropivacaine [6], or adjuvants [7] to an opioid improved analgesic efficacy and reduced the dose requirements for either drug alone. Moreover, bupivacaine–morphine combination presented more effective neuropathic pain relief, and there was no neurotoxicity in long-term infusion than morphine alone [8].

Clonidine decreases the pain transmission, miming inhibitory descending bulbospinal neurons, through the stimulation of α2-receptors in the dorsal horn. This drug also potentiates sensory and motor blockade of epidural and peripheral nerve block with local anesthetics blocking the conduction in C and Aδ fibers, through *cholinergic* mechanisms, and causing local vasoconstriction. Also, ketamine in small doses is helpful in pain relief [9]. However, there is insufficient evidence to recommend one drug option or regimen over another [5].

By reason of epidural, opioid administration reaches the receptor in two ways: by the systemic absorption and by the penetration of the dura mater and the arachnoid; plasma opioid concentrations after epidural administration are similar to plasma opioid concentrations after intramuscular injections when using lipophilic agents such as sufentanil. Thus, the risk of systemic opioid side effects after epidural administration is higher than in intrathecal administration [10].

Infection is a major problem associated with catheter use. In a systemic review of 24 studies, Ruppen et al. [11] reported that catheter-related infection was superficial (4.6 %) and deep (1.2 %). They pointed that the infection may more easily occur with long term of catheter insertion and when the latter has no subcutaneous tunneling.

Table 7.1 shows the afferent innervation and spinal cord localization of the pelvic viscera. Indications and contraindications of epidural analgesia in cancer patient are shown in Table 7.2, while in Table 7.3 recommendations developed by the American Society of Regional Anesthesia and Pain Medicine (ASRA) for patients taking anticoagulants are reported [12].

TABLE 7.1. Afferent innervation and spinal cord localization of the pelvic viscera and perineum

Organ	Spinal innervation	Sympathetic and peripheral nerves
Ovary	T10, T11, T12	Renal/aortic plexus
Testes	T10, T11, T12	Renal/aortic plexus
Vas deferens, epididymis	T10, T11, T12, L1	Renal/aortic plexus
Spermatic cord, tunica vaginalis	L1, L2	Genital branch genitofemoral nerve
Uterus	T10, T11, T12, L1	Superior hypogastric plexus (presacral nerve)
Bladder and uterers, superior vagina, inferior portion of uterine segment	T10, T11, T12, L1-5, (S2–4)	Superior hypogastric plexus (presacral nerve), inferior hypogastric plexus, inguinal, genitofemoral nerve
Distal colon and rectum	T10, T11, T12, L1-5, S2–4	Superior hypogastric plexus (presacral nerve), inferior hypogastric plexus, inguinal, genitofemoral nerve

(continued)

TABLE 7.1 (continued)

Organ	Spinal innervation	Sympathetic and peripheral nerves
Cervix	T10, T11, T12, L1	Superior hypogastric plexus (presacral nerve)
Proximal fallopian tubes	T10, T11, T12, L1	Superior hypogastric plexus (presacral nerve) (Celiac plexus)
Distal fallopian tubes	T10, T11, T12	Renal/aortic plexus (ovarian plexus)
Broad ligaments	T10, T11	Renal/aortic plexus
Renal pelvis, ureter	T10, T11, T12, L1	Renal plexus
Bladder neck	S2-4	Inferior hypogastric plexus
Lower vagina, vulva, perineum	(T12), L1-5, S2–4	Pudendal nerve, Iliohypogastric nerve, Ilio-inguinal nerve, genitofemoral nerve, Ganglion Impair

TABLE 7.2. Epidural analgesia in cancer patient

Indications	Contraindications
[a]**A high pain score pain despite aggressive pharmacologic interventions by conventional administration routes (oral, rectal, transdermal, subcutaneous, and intravenous)** **Continuous intermittent and intermittent pain patterns** **Intractable severe or dose-limiting side effects experienced from conventional administration route** **Patient acceptance**	Platelets count <20,000 Oral anticoagulant therapy (see Table 7.3) International normalized ratio ≥1.5 Active local infection or concurrent septicemia Occlusion of the epidural space or myelopathy Increased intracranial pressure Patient refusal

[a]In patients with an acceptable life expectancy (more than 3 months?) consider the continuous intrathecal infusion, if there are no serious contraindications, such as respiratory insufficiency or sleep apnea, altered consciousness and psychological disorders, patients who are hemodynamically unstable or have spinal cord pathology with cerebrospinal fluid outflow obstruction, intracranial hypertension, sepsis or infection at the site of the catheter or pump insertion

TABLE 7.3. ASRA's consensus statement on Regional Anesthesia in the Anticoagulated Patient [12]

Drug	Catheter insertion	Catheter removal
NSAIDs	No contraindication; may increase frequency of spontaneous hemorrhagic complications when combined with warfarin, heparin, or thrombolytics	No contraindication
Ticlopidine	Discontinue 14 days before insertion	
Clopidogrel	Discontinue 7 days before insertion	
GP IIb/IIIa inhibitorsa	Discontinue 8–48 h before insertion	
Heparin	SC/IV: Do not heparinize until at least 1 h after the epidural block IV infusion: Discontinue heparin infusion for 2–4 h and check partial thromboplastin (PTT) prior to block	Wait 2–4 h after last SC heparin dose or discontinuing IV heparin infusion; check PTT prior to removal
Warfarin	Discontinue 4–5 days prior to neuraxial manipulation; INR should be normal prior to block	May remove catheter when INR is ≤1.5 after discontinuing warfarin
Low molecular weight heparin (LMWH)b	Wait for 12–24 h after the last dose	Remove 2 h prior LMWH dose
Thrombolyticsc	Data limited; follow fibrinogen levels; original contraindications called for avoidance of drugs for 10 days following puncture of noncompressible vessels	No definite recommendations; measure fibrinogen level to help decide between catheter removal or maintenance

(continued)

TABLE 7.3 (continued)

Drug	Catheter insertion	Catheter removal
Herbals	No definitive recommendations; watch for "3 Gs" (ginseng, garlic, ginkgo biloba) that are known to either have antiplatelet properties or enhance effect of antiplatelet drugs	

[a]GP IIb/IIIa inhibitors include tirofiban, eptifibatide, abciximab
[b]LMWHs include ardeparin, dalteparin, danaparoid, enoxaparin, and tinzaparin
[c]Thrombolytics include urokinase, streptokinase, endogenous t-PA formulations

7.2   Intrathecal Drug Delivery

Since the first reservoir for intrathecal medications was implanted in 1981 [13], several experiences have declared intrathecal drug delivery (IDD) therapy as a safe and effective route of administration for medications used to treat intractable pain and spasticity [14] in appropriately selected patients [15, 16]. Thus, IDD can be used to deliver multiple medications, such as morphine, baclofen, local anesthetics (bupivacaine hydrochloride), clonidine, and ziconotide [17] directly into the intrathecal space of the spine.

Although this is an invasive technique, it provides a good pain relief with just a small amount of medication and few side effects in cancer and non-cancer patients. Indeed, studies showed the positive results of the application of IDD in advanced cancer patients who were highly opioid tolerant and previously treated with multiple opioid trials unsuccessfully [18].

There are several devices for delivering medications intrathecally. They use external pumps with a percutaneous catheter (tunneled or not tunneled) or fully implantable devices

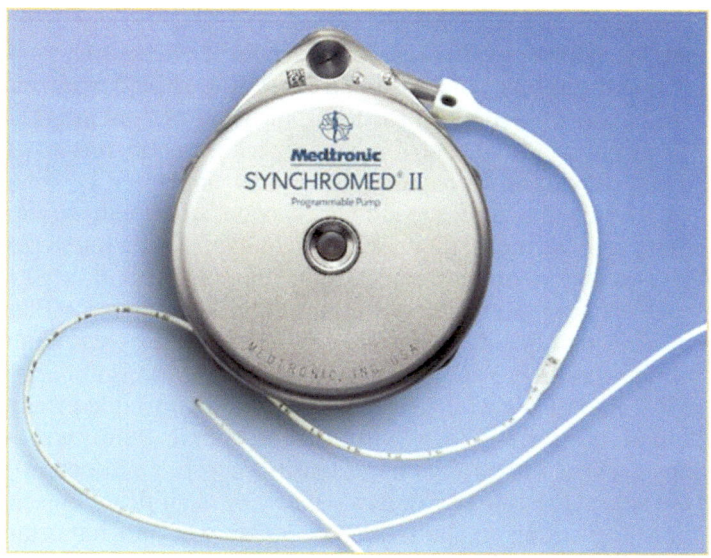

FIGURE 7.1. Fully implanted intrathecal pump (Courtesy from Medtronic®)

(subcutaneous injection port or small pumps inserted under the skin, usually in abdomen). Among these, there are fully implanted programmable IDD devices (Fig. 7.1) in which dose changes are quite useful for conditions such as opioid tolerance or dynamic changes in pain that necessitate frequent dose alterations for patients with cancer. Bolus doses can be given by programming the pump to give doses at set times and, when available, by giving the patient the option of delivering boluses as needed, a concept known as patient-controlled analgesia (PCA), which may be achieved with a personal therapy manager (PTM). In most cases, the PTM is set to give 5–20 % of the daily dose that is administered at the continuous rate [19].

The continuous intrathecal infusion was initially indicated in patients with long life expectancy which are not responders to the traditional pharmacological approaches [20, 21]. However, the Polyanalgesic Consensus Committee (PACC) stated, in 2012, that life expectancy may be increased with intrathecal therapy because of reduced side effects, suggesting that in the absence of impending death IDD should be considered even if a patient's prognosis falls short of 3 months [22]. The same asserted that for patients with a short life expectancy, percutaneous catheter (or totally implanted catheters with a subcutaneous injection port) connected to an external pump may be more suitable, instead of implantable pump [23].

The continuous intrathecal infusion is contraindicated in patients who are unable/unwilling to have the pump refilled or have significant coagulopathies which require therapeutic anticoagulation. Yet, this route of administration is not applicable in patients who are hemodynamically unstable or have spinal cord pathology with cerebrospinal fluid outflow obstruction, intracranial hypertension, sepsis, an infection at the site of the catheter or pump insertion, significant emaciation preventing implantation of the device, and important psychiatric comorbidities [23].

Among the IDD complications, we report the possibility of respiratory depression, post-dural puncture headaches, dislocations of the catheters, and formation of granulomas. According to the PACC, the latter complication can be prevented by the use of the lowest effective dose and concentration of intrathecal opioids or using an intermittent bolus dosing. Furthermore, the use of ziconotide or fentanyl does not seem to lead to this complication [22]. Low starting doses of opioids are also recommended to avoid the risk of respiratory depression.

Epidural infusion requires substantial dosages, high volumes, and more frequently refills when compared to intrathecal catheters resulting in higher costs and infection rates. While persistent nausea, persistent and transient urinary retention, transient pruritus, and constipation occurred more frequently with epidural infusion, respiratory depression, sedation, and confusion were most common with intrathecal catheters [24].

It is difficult to respond to the question on which is the more effective and safe type of central neuraxial blocks usable to treat pelvic cancer pain when pharmacological approaches failed. We suggest a strong case-by-case analysis. For instance, in a patient with a stabilized disease, and with an acceptable life expectancy (more than 3 months?), we prefer a continuous intrathecal infusion, if there are no serious contraindications (see Table 7.2 *notes*). Comorbidity, such as sleep apnea, or other respiratory conditions discourage the choice of IDD. Peripheral edema is also a relative limitation, as it is sometimes associated with the use of intrathecal opioid therapy with a mechanism related to an effect of these agents on the levels of antidiuretic hormone [25]. On the other hand, epidural analgesia is easy to perform and is effective for patients with a short predicted survival. Moreover, it does not require trained operators and expensive, and not always available, devices.

Suggestions for Conversion from Systemic to Epidural/Spinal Morphine

- 300 mg oral morphine = 100 mg parenteral = 10 mg epidural = 1 mg intrathecal
- 50% dose chosen may be given systemically and slowly reduced to 20% per day to prevent possible withdrawal symptoms

Intrathecal Drug Delivery

- Recommended boli trialing: morphine 0.2–1.0 mg, hydromorphone 0.04–0.2 mg, ziconotide 1–5 mcg, fentanyl 25–75 mcg, bupivacaine 0.5–2.5 mg, clonidine 5–20 mcg, and sufentanil 5–20 mcg [22]
- Maximum dose per day: morphine 15 mg, hydromorphone 10 mg, bupivacaine 10 mg, clonidine 40–600 mcg, and ziconotide 19.2 mcg [22]

References

1. Chambers WA (2008) Nerve blocks in palliative care. Br J Anaesth 101(1):95–100
2. Hogan Q, Haddox JD, Abram S et al (1991) Epidural opiates and local anesthetics for the management of cancer pain. Pain 46:271–279
3. Smitt PS, Tsafka A, Teng-van de Zande F et al (1998) Outcome and complications of epidural analgesia in patients with chronic cancer pain. Cancer 83:2015–2022
4. van Dongen RT, Crul BJ, van Egmond J (1999) Intrathecal coadministration of bupivacaine diminishes morphine dose progression during long-term intrathecal infusion in cancer patients. Clin J Pain 15(3):166–172
5. Dahm P, Lundborg C, Janson M et al (2000) Comparison of 0.5% intrathecal bupivacaine with 0.5% intrathecal ropivacaine in the treatment of refractory cancer and non cancer pain conditions: results from a prospective, crossover, double-blind, randomized study. Reg Anesth Pain Med 25(5):480–487
6. Lauretti GR, Gomes JM, Reis MP et al (1999) Low doses of epidural ketamine or neostigmine, but not midazolam, improve morphine analgesia in epidural terminal cancer pain therapy. J Clin Anesth 11(8):663–668
7. Sjöberg M, Karlsson PA, Nordborg C (1992) Neuropathologic findings after long-term intrathecal infusion of morphine and bupivacaine for pain treatment in cancer patients. Anesthesiology 76:173–186
8. Congedo E, Sgreccia M, De Cosmo G (2009) New drugs for epidural analgesia. Curr Drug Targets 10:696–706
9. Myers J, Chan V, Jarvis V et al (2010) Intraspinal techniques for pain management in cancer patients: a systematic review. Support Care Cancer 18(2):137–149
10. Wagemans MF, Zuurmond WW, de Lange JJ (1997) Long-term spinal opioid therapy in terminally ill cancer pain patients. Oncologist 2(2):70–75
11. Ruppen W, Derry S, McQuay HJ et al (2007) Infection rates associated with epidural indwelling catheters for seven days or longer: systematic review and meta-analysis. BMC Palliat Care 6:3
12. Horlocker TT, Wedel DJ, Rowlingson JC et al (2010) Regional anesthesia in the patient receiving antithrombotic or thrombolytic therapy: American Society of Regional Anesthesia and Pain

Medicine Evidence-Based Guidelines (Third Edition) Conference on Neuraxial Anesthesia and Anticoagulation. Reg Anesth Pain Med 35(1):64–101

13. Onofrio BM, Yaksh TL, Arnold PG (1981) Continuous low-dose intrathecal morphine administration in the treatment of chronic pain of malignant origin. Mayo Clin Proc 56:516–520

14. Ontario HQ (2005) Intrathecal baclofen pump for spasticity: an evidence-based analysis. Ont Health Technol Assess Ser 5(7):1–93

15. Rauck R, Deer T, Rosen S (2010) Accuracy and efficacy of intrathecal administration of morphine sulfate for treatment of intractable pain using the Prometra(®) Programmable Pump. Neuromodulation 13(2):102–108

16. Rauck R, Deer T, Rosen S (2013) Long-term follow-up of a novel implantable programmable infusion pump. Neuromodulation 16(2):163–167

17. Ellis DJ, Dissanayake S, McGuire D et al (2008) Continuous intrathecal infusion of ziconotide for treatment of chronic malignant and nonmalignant pain over 12 months: a prospective, open-label study. Neuromodulation 11(1):40–49

18. Mercadante S, Intravaia G, Villari P et al (2007) Intrathecal treatment in cancer patients unresponsive to multiple trials of systemic opioids. Clin J Pain 23(9):793–798

19. Perruchoud C, Eldabe S, Durrer A (2011) Effects of flow rate modifications on reported analgesia and quality of life in chronic pain patients treated with continuous intrathecal drug therapy. Pain Med 12:571–576

20. Smith TJ, Staats PS, Deer T, Implantable Drug Delivery Systems Study Group (2002) Randomized clinical trial of an implantable drug delivery system compared with comprehensive medical management for refractory cancer pain: impact on pain, drug related toxicity and survival. J Clin Oncol 20:4040–4049

21. Christo PJ, Mazloomdoost D (2008) Interventional pain treatments for cancer pain. Ann N Y Acad Sci 1138:299–328

22. Deer TR, Prager J, Levy R et al (2012) Polyanalgesic consensus conference 2012: recommendations for the management of pain by intrathecal (intraspinal) drug delivery: Report of an interdisciplinary expert panel. Neuromodulation 15:436–464

23. Smith TJ, Coyne PJ (2003) How to use implantable intrathecal drug delivery systems for refractory cancer pain. J Support Oncol 1:73–76

24. Ballantyne JC, Carwood CM (2005) Comparative efficacy of epidural, subarachnoid, and intracerebroventricular opioids in patients with pain due to cancer. Cochrane Database Syst Rev (1):CD005178. doi: 10.1002/14651858

25. Paice JA, Penn RD, Shott S (1996) Intraspinal morphine for chronic pain: a retrospective, multicenter study. J Pain Symptom Manage 11:71–80

Chapter 8
Neurolytic Sympathetic Plexus Blocks

Pain from malignant involvement of visceral organs is conveyed along sympathetic pathways and may be amenable to interruption of these pathways [1] (see also Table 7.1).

Neurolytic block is recommended only when opioids fail to control the pain, when the side effects of systemic pharmacotherapy become too debilitating [2], or to control intractable pain associated with involvement of nerves or plexi. However, some authors have proposed the application of these procedures in the beginning stages of cancer pain management for preventing the development of pain and improving the QoL of patients, also in pelvic cancer pain. For instance, de Olivera et al. demonstrated both a significant reduction of pain and opioid consumption in patients who received neurolytic sympathetic plexus block compared with those treated by pharmacological therapy only [3]. Among the advantages, these nerve blocks can sometimes be given as a series of several injections, repeated at weekly intervals. On the other hand, the availability of trained staff and the lack of precise criteria are significant limits in their spread for cancer pain management. There is no consensus, indeed, about the optimum technique, interval between blocks, and duration of treatment. Moreover, although these approaches could be effective in visceral pain, the results in terms of pain relief have been less tangible for neuropathic pain, as it is often multifactorial and not completely abolished by sympatholysis. However, the literature shows that there may be evidence for

© Springer International Publishing Switzerland 2016
M. Cascella et al., *Features and Management of the Pelvic Cancer Pain*, DOI 10.1007/978-3-319-33587-2_8

the role of sympathetic blocks in management of cancer pain (also pelvic cancer pain) [4], rather than their effectiveness for reducing pain in nonmalignant conditions, such as post-herpetic neuralgia, low back pain, and complex regional pain syndrome [5]. These observations suggest to consider also neurolytic sympathetic plexus blocks as a component of multimodal pain management strategy. Thus, although not as first choice, in selected patients, sympatholysis could represent an effective strategy when pain is resistant to or when intolerable adverse effects preclude the use of traditional pharmacotherapeutics, as well as when it is not possible to resort to central neuraxial blocks. For this purpose, neurolytic blocks could allow a significant reduction in opioids usage, improving the QoL.

As contraindications of neurolytic blocks, we indicate patient refusal, bleeding diatheses, and infection at the site of injection. About the anticoagulant therapy, we usually follow the recommendations developed for perioperative management of patients who are receiving anticoagulant or antiplatelet drugs and require surgical or invasive procedure, assessing the thromboembolic and the bleeding risks [6].

In pelvic cancer pain, there are several techniques to perform neurolytic sympathetic plexus blocks, including the most common used superior hypogastric plexus block, the inferior hypogastric plexus block, the neurolysis of the Ganglion Impar, and the presacral plexus neurolytic block. Sympatholysis is usually performed with local anesthetics or neurolytics (phenol and alcohol).

8.1   Superior Hypogastric Plexus Block

Hypogastric blocks may be useful in the treatment of chronic pelvic pain, especially of neoplastic origin [7]. Patients with pain due to cervical, endometrial, prostatic, testicular, and colorectal cancer have been treated with Superior Hypogastric Plexus Block (SHPB) and success (VAS < 4 and significant reductions in opioids dosage) appears to occur in 70 %, until patient's demise [8].

The superior hypogastric plexus is located in the retroperitoneum in correspondence of the lower third of the body of the 5th lumbar vertebra (L5) and the upper third of the body of the 1st sacral (S1) at the sacral promontory, on the midline just caudal to the bifurcation of the common iliac vessels. It is formed by pelvis visceral afferents and efferent sympathetic nerves from branches of the aortic plexus and fibers from the splanchnic nerves. On this plexus converge hypogastric nerves that carry afferents from the pelvic viscera; indeed, its location allows it to innervate the vast majority of pelvic viscera, including the bladder, urethra, uterus, vagina, vulva, perineum, prostate, penis, testes, rectum, and descending colon.

The SHPB can be done as posterior approach (classic posterolateral approach or transdiscal in prone position), anterior approach (supine position), or lateral approach (transdiscal) (Fig. 8.1). The classic posterolateral percutaneous approach has been described by Plancarte et al. [9], in 1990, as an evolution of the Cotte's presacral neurectomy [10]. In a large cohort study, Plancarte et al. [11] showed that this block provided both effective pain relief and a significant reduction in opioid usage (43 %) in 72 % of the patients. Under fluoroscopy guide, the posterior approach involves a percutaneous insertion, in the prone position with a pillow beneath the pelvis to reduce the lumbar lordosis, of two 22-Gauge (G) 6-in. needles (one for each side) from 5 cm lateral the L5 spinous process toward midline (30° caudal and 45° medially), until the anterior lateral region of the intervertebral space L5/S1. After verification of the position by injection of 3–4 ml of radio-opaque contrast (the contrast should spread toward the midline from the bilaterally placed paramedian sites), 6–8 ml bupivacaine 0.25 for testing block procedures can be used. For therapeutic purposes, 5–8 ml of 10 % aqueous phenol, or 15–30 ml of ethanol [3], at each side of the vertebra can be used.

With this approach, the iliac crest and L5 transverse process are potential anatomical barriers to proper needle placement; moreover, often there is the patient's inability to lie in prone position.

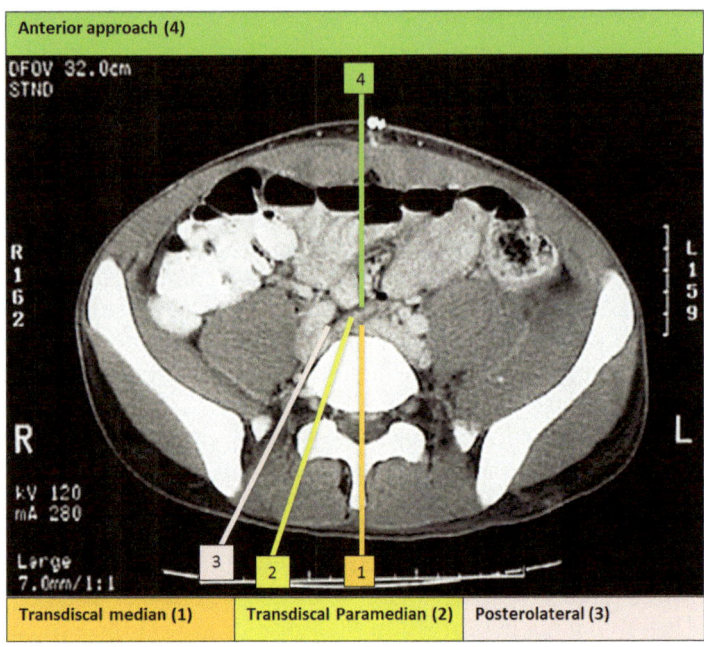

FIGURE 8.1. Different approaches for neurolytic superior hypogastric plexus block under CT guide (1–3 posterior approaches; 4 anterior approach; 2 also as lateral approach)

Several investigators reported good results using a paramedian or posteromedian transdiscal approach with a single puncture and performed with the patient in either lateral or prone position [12–14]. In paramedian discal approach, entry point is again 5–7 cm from the midline at L5–S1 but introduced just lateral to the inferior aspect of the facet joint and advanced through the disk under lateral fluoroscopic guidance, till loss of resistance is felt. In posteromedian approach, needle is inserted perpendicularly to the skin at the center of the L5–S1 interlaminar space under anteroposterior fluoroscopic vision. The needle is then advanced toward the intervertebral disk so that it penetrates the thecal sac under lateral fluoroscopic control.

The transdiscal approach is associated with a potential disk rupture, disk herniation, or discitis. The literature quotes <5 % rate of post-procedural discitis [12] though several studies have suggested that the use of preoperative intravenous or injection of antibiotics into the disk during transdiscal approaches may prevent this complication [15–17].

A more recent attempt for the SHPB is the anterior approach. It is applicable in patients who may not be able to lie prone, or when posterior and transdiscal approaches are not suitable for anatomical difficulties, such as osteophytic overgrowth, or in the presence of radiculopathy or disk diseases. As first described by Kanazi in 1999 [18], with the patient placed in supine Trendeleburg position (15°), and after infiltration with local anesthetic of an area 2–5 cm inferior the umbilicus, a 22-G 6-in. needle is inserted toward the inferior two-thirds the L5 vertebral body until the bony contact. The angular of the approach is perpendicular to the floor, and a continuous aspiration is necessary to identify accidental visceral or vascular penetration. After fluoroscopic confirmation by injection of radio-opaque contrast, a solution of 20–30 ml of 0.25 % of bupivacaine followed by phenol or alcohol is injected for neurolysis. This is a fascinating approach; nevertheless, in accordance with Gupta [19], it may expose the patient to a higher risk of bowel perforation, ureteral damage, and infection, also when performed under computed tomography [20] or ultrasound guide [21]. It is imperative that bladder is empty and patient receives pre-procedure antibiotics as traversing small/large bowel is inevitable.

Several authors assume that the risks for the neurolytic block of the superior hypogastric plexus are low, especially when performed under CT guide [22]. Intravenous fluid is recommended pre- and post-procedure because of the risk of hypotension (30 %) within first 12 h of procedure due to loss of sympathetic tone and splanchnic vasodilatation, while common complications include transient pain from the procedure and diarrhea (60 %, but resolving within 48 h). However, the procedure may result in neurological complications (paraplegia, leg weakness, sensory deficits, and paresthesia due to direct injury to spinal cord or injection into anterior spinal artery), vascular injury, or chemical peritonitis. Chan et al. [23] described a patient developing somatic nerve damage after a computed tomography scan-guided neurolytic block; however, they pointed out that the patient's severe kyphoscoliotic lumbosacral junction deformity and his semi-recumbent position may have contributed to the development of the complication. In spite of this report, in Plancarte's study, no neurological complications were detected following this neurolytic block [11], but the theoretical risks of this procedure exist, including cerebrospinal fluid leak, intrathecal or epidural injection, bleeding, especially into retroperitoneal space, nerve injury and/or paralysis with transient bowel, bladder and sexual dysfunction, and puncture of surrounding organs or vessels. De Leon-Casasola also described the possibility of distal ischemia due to puncture of the iliac artery, as well as the risks of systemic complications if the medication is injected into a blood vessel, and the risk of infection [24].

Summarizing, bowel, bladder, and ureteral damages are mainly related to the anterior approach, while, given the proximity of vascular structures, the posterior approach exposes the patient to risk of bleeding and hematoma, and the transdiscal approach is associated with a disk damage and infection. Although, all these risks could be reduced using a computed tomography or ultrasound guide (anterior approach), fluoroscopy tends to be the preferred imaging method.

8.2   Inferior Hypogastric Plexus Block

Despite the comforting initial data using SHPB, some authors have reported poor results in patients with extensive retroperitoneal disease overlying the plexus, as well as in patients presenting with low pelvic pain combined with perineal pain (anal pain or pain arising from the genitalia). In these cases, the quality of evidence of SHPB, according to scoring system published by Van Zundert et al., is only 2 C+ (benefits closely balanced with risks; considered, preferably study related)

[25]. These observations led to a better study of the function and the anatomy of the inferior hypogastric plexus. This plexus is the primary autonomic neural coordinating center in the pelvis through which most nociceptive information will pass. It integrates both parasympathetic and sympathetic output and receives input from the sacral level of the spinal cord. The plexus is formed by efferent sympathetic fibers from the hypogastric nerves and from pelvic splanchnic nerves, supplying branches to the pelvic viscera directly, as well as from subsidiary plexuses (e.g., the superior, middle rectal, bladder, prostate, and uterovaginal plexuses). It also receives preganglionic parasympathetic fibers from pelvic splanchnic nerves and visceral afferent fibers from pelvic viscera [26–28]. For these reasons, according to Mohamed et al. [29], the Inferior Hypogastric Plexus Block (IHPB) can better realize the pain control in extensive cancer diseases, reducing the opioids dosage in cancer patients presenting with low pelvic pain combined with perineal pain, namely, anal pain, or pain arising from the genitalia. However, this plexus is not easily assessable to blockade by local anesthetics and neurolytic agents. Schultz's neurolytic IHPB via transsacral approach has several disadvantages because of transient paresthesia, nerve damage, rectal puncture, vascular penetration, hematoma, and infection [30] and requires expertise of the operator. Although other authors reported a safely fluoroscopy-guided IHPB via coccygeal transverse approach [31], the risk of complications, as rectal trauma, is high.

8.3 Neurolysis of the Ganglion Impar

Visceral pain in the perineal area associated with malignancies may be effectively treated with neurolysis of the Ganglion Impar. This ganglion (also known as the ganglion of Walther) is a solitary anatomical feature, found on the ventral surface of the coccyx, at the level of the sacrococcygeal joint, where it forms the caudal origin of the bilateral sympathetic chain, indeed. It provides sympathetic innervation to the perineum, distal rectum, anus, distal urethra, vulva, coccyx, scrotum, and distal third of the vagina.

First described by Plancarte et al. in 1990 [32], the block technique was performed with the patient in the prone position using fluoroscopic guidance and a manually bent 22 G spinal needle directed cephalad through the anococcygeal ligaments. The needle is then advanced until the tip is placed posterior to the rectum.

This block may be performed with the patient in the left lateral decubitus position with the knees flexed, in the lithotomy position. Moreover, a trans-sacrococcygeal approach to a Ganglion Impar block, described by Wemm and Saberski in 1995, was developed to improve the technical feasibility and overcome the associated risk for visceral injuries with a conventional technique [33]. More recently, the Plancarte's original technique has been extensively modified by Gupta et al. [34] who described an easy and safe ultrasound-guided improvement.

Neurolytic block of the Ganglion Impar, producing prolonged disruption of afferent sympathetic and nociceptive routes from the pelvis and perineal/anal area, is effectively used in otherwise difficult cases with a highly desirable risk-to-benefit ratio [35]. Recently, some authors described a SHPB, by a posteromedian transdiscal approach, combined with a Ganglion Impar neurolytic block through a trans-sacrococcygeal approach using a 22-G 2 in. needle and injection of 4–6 ml of 8 % phenol in saline. They found a reduction in pain scores and in consumption of oral morphine after the first 24 h post-procedure in 66.6 % of patients, with no complications or serious side effects. They recorded only transient paresthesia and pain on injection [36].

8.4   Presacral Plexus Neurolytic Block

The sacral plexus (plexus sacralis) is a nerve plexus which is formed by anterior rami of L4 to S5, providing motor and sensory nerves for the posterior thigh, most of the lower leg and foot, and part of the pelvis. It lies on the back of the pelvis between the piriformis muscle and the pelvic fascia.

According to Wilsey [37], this block could be useful for the treatment of unrelieved pelvic and perineal pain in advanced cancer. Although the author described an easy and safety technique — performed with a lateral CT guided approach — there are few data in the literature to confirm and validate the procedure.

Are sympathetic blocks really effective for pelvic cancer pain management? In a recent systematic review on sympathetic blocks for visceral cancer pain management [38], the authors found only one controlled study, performed in patients with pelvic cancer pain associated with gynecological cancer [39]. Although in this study patients treated with the block (SHPB by anterior approach) had a decrease in pain intensity and a smaller morphine consumption, the authors of the review stated that the quality of the investigation was very poor due to several limitations, including sample size calculation, allocation concealment, and no intention to treat analysis [38]. Moreover, because somatic pain and neuropathic pain often coexist and mixed syndromes are more likely to be observed in patients with pelvic tumors than in those with abdominal pain, interruption of sympathetic pathway is not a guarantee for abolishing all types of pain inputs [38]. Consequently, sympathetic procedures for pain conditions due to pelvic cancers should be intended as adjuvant techniques, for instance, with the purpose of reducing the analgesic consumption [39]. Additionally, sympathetic blocks can be used for diagnostic purposes in order to determine if the pain is sympathetically mediated or not.

Practical Suggestion

Because pelvic cancer pain is not the result of a pure visceral mechanism, according to the EAPC recommendations, neurolytic sympathetic blocks should be performed not as first choice, but only after a thorough case-by-case analysis.

Limitations: availability of trained staff and the lack of precise criteria.

References

1. De Leon-Casasola OA (2000) Critical evaluation of chemical neurolysis of the sympathetic axis for cancer pain. Cancer Control 7(2):142–148

2. Caraceni A, Portenoy RK (1996) Pain management in patients with pancreatic carcinoma. Cancer 78(3 Suppl):639–653

3. de Oliveira R, dos Reisa MP, Pradob WA (2004) The effects of early or late neurolytic sympathetic plexus block on the management of abdominal or pelvic cancer pain. Pain 110(1–2): 400–408

4. Boas RA (1998) Sympathetic nerve blocks: in search of a role. Reg Anesth Pain Med 23:292–305

5. Stanton TR, Wand BM, Carr DB et al (2013) Local anaesthetic sympathetic blockade for complex regional pain syndrome. Cochrane Database Syst Rev 8, CD004598. doi:10.1002/14651858. CD004598.pub3

6. Cuomo A, Cascella M, Bifulco F et al (2015) Periprocedural management of antithrombotic therapy and open issues in cancer patients. Minerva Anestesiol 81(11):1229–1243

7. Vissers KC, Besse K, Wagemans M (2011) Pain in patients with cancer. Pain Pract 11:453–475

8. De Leon-Casasola OA, Kent E, Lema MJ (1993) Neurolytic superior hypogastric plexus block for chronic pelvic pain associated with cancer. Pain 54(2):145–151

9. Plancarte R, Amescua C, Patt RB (1990) Superior hypogastric plexus block for pelvic cancer pain. Anesthesiology 73(2): 236–239

10. Cotte MG (1925) Sur le traitement des dysmenorrhees rebelles par la sympathectomie hypogastrique periaterielle ou la section du nerf presacre. Lyon Med 6:135–153

11. Plancarte R, de Leon-Casasola OA, El-Helaly M (1997) Neurolytic superior hypogastric plexus block for chronic pelvic pain associated with cancer. Reg Anesth 22(6):562–568

12. Erdine S, Yucel A, Celik M et al (2003) Transdiscal approach for hypogastric plexus block. Reg Anesth Pain Med 28(4):304–308

13. Turker G, Basagan-Mogol E, Gurbet A (2005) A new technique for superior hypogastric plexus block: the posteromedian transdiscal approach. Tohoku J Exp Med 206(3):277–281

14. Nabil D, Eissa AA (2010) Evaluation of posteromedial transdiscal superior hypogastric block after failure of the classic approach. Clin J Pain 26(8):694–697

15. Fraser R, Osti O, Vernon-Roberts B (1989) Iatrogenic discitis: the role of intravenous antibiotics in prevention and treatment. An experimental study. Spine 14:1025–1032

16. Walters R, Moore R, Fraser R (2006) Penetration of cephazolin in human lumbar intervertebral disc. Spine 31:567–570

17. Walters R, Rahmat R, Shimamura Y et al (2006) Prophylactic cephazolin to prevent discitis in an ovine model. Spine 31:391–396

18. Kanazi GE, Perkins FM, Thakur R et al (1999) New technique for superior hypogastric plexus block. Reg Anesth Pain Med 24(5):473–476

19. Gupta A (ed) (2012) Interventional pain medicine. Oxford University Press, New York

20. Michalek P, Dutka J (2005) Computed tomography-guided anterior approach to the superior hypogastric plexus for noncancer pelvic pain: a report of two cases. Clin J Pain 21(6):553–556

21. Mishra S, Bhatnagar S, Gupta D (2008) Anterior ultrasound-guided superior hypogastric plexus neurolysis in pelvic cancer pain. Anaesth Intensive Care 36(5):732–735

22. Ghoneim AA, Mansour SM (2014) Comparative study between computed tomography guided superior hypogastric plexus block and the classic posterior approach: a prospective randomized study. Saudi J Anaesth 8(3):378–383

23. Chan WS, Peh WC, Ng KF et al (1997) Computed tomography scan-guided neurolytic superior hypogastric block complicated by somatic nerve damage in a severely kyphoscoliotic patient. Anesthesiology 86(6):1429–1430

24. De Leon-Casasola O, Molloy RE, Lema M (2005) Neurolytic visceral sympathetic blocks. In: Benzon HT, Raja SN, Molloy RE et al (eds) Essentials of pain medicine and regional anesthesia, 2nd edn. Elsevier-Churchill Livingston, New York, pp 542–549

25. Van Zundert J, Hartrick C, Patijn J (2011) Evidence-based interventional pain medicine according to clinical diagnoses. Pain Pract 11:423–429

26. Christo J, Hobelmann G (2009) Pelvic pain. In: Smith HS (ed) Current therapy in pain, 1st edn. Saunders-Elsevier, Philadelphia, PA, pp 216–227

27. Waldman S (2009) Hypogastric plexus block. In: Waldman SD (ed) Pain review, 1st edn. Saunders-Elsevier, Philadelphia, PA, pp 538–541

28. Waldman S (2004) Atlas of interventional pain management. Saunders, Philadelphia, PA

29. Mohamed SA, Ahmed DG, Mohamad MF (2013) Chemical neurolysis of the inferior hypogastric plexus for the treatment of cancer-related pelvic and perineal pain. Pain Res Manage 18:249–252
30. Schultz DM (2007) Inferior hypogastric plexus blockade: a transsacral approach. Pain Physician 10:757–763
31. Choi HS, Kim YH, Han JW et al (2012) A new technique for inferior hypogastric plexus block: a coccygeal transverse approach—a case report. Korean J Pain 25(1):38–42
32. Plancarte R, Amescua C, Patt RB et al (1990) Presacral blockade of the ganglion of Walter (ganglion impar). Anesthesiology 73(3A):A751
33. Wemm K, Saberski L (1995) Modified approach to block the ganglion impar (ganglion of Walther). Reg Anesth 20:544–545
34. Gupta D, Jain R, Mishra S et al (2008) Ultrasonography reinvents the originally described technique for ganglion impar neurolysis in perianal cancer pain. Anesth Analg 107(4):1390–1392
35. Malec-Milewska M, Horosz B, Kolęda I et al (2014) Neurolytic block of ganglion of Walther for the management of chronic pelvic pain. Wideochir Inne Tech Maloinwazyjne 9(3):458–462
36. Ahmed DG, Mohamed MF, Mohamed SA (2015) Superior hypogastric plexus combined with ganglion impar neurolytic blocks for pelvic and/or perineal cancer pain relief. Pain Physician 18(1):E49–E56
37. Wilsey C, Ashford NS, Dolin SJ (2002) Presacral neurolytic blocks for relief of pain from pelvic cancer: description and use of CT guided lateral approach. Palliat Med 16:441–444
38. Mercadante S, Klepstad P, Kurita GP, European Palliative Care Research Collaborative (EPCRC) (2015) Sympathetic blocks for visceral cancer pain management: a systematic review and EAPC recommendations. Crit Rev Oncol Hematol 96(3):577–583
39. Mishra S, Bhatnagar S, Rana SP et al (2013) Efficacy of the anterior ultrasound-guided superior hypogastric plexus neurolysis in pelvic cancer pain in advanced gynecological cancer patients. Pain Med 14:837–842

Chapter 9
Minimally Invasive Palliative Treatments

A special chapter of pain management in patients affected by refractory cancer pain, not responding to "standard" treatments, concerns the possibility of using MIPPs [1]. This term refers to several techniques based on the use of percutaneous image-guided methods to deliver tissue ablative materials or devices inside the neoplastic lesion (see also our review on the topic in the American Journal of Hospice and Palliative Medicine, *in press*). Vertebral osteolytic metastasis, for instance, is more commonly treated using percutaneous vertebroplasty or percutaneous balloon kyphoplasty with an excellent long-term palliation of pain and improving mobility and QoL [2]. MIPPs are mostly used also for painful metastatic disease as well as in nonsurgical pelvic recurrence of cancer. These non-pharmacological approaches can not only be used to treat cancer lesions, such as metastases or local recurrences, but also to perform techniques of neurolysis in pelvic pain secondary to malignancy. For instance, the blockade of Ganglion Impar can be obtained also by cryoablation [3] or radiofrequency ablation (RFA) [4].

In pelvic cancer diseases, a key concept regards the indications of MIPPs. These percutaneous treatments should be considered if the patient has pain not controllable by narcotic analgesics or not responding to earlier applied therapies and is not eligible for a surgical resection due to advanced disease and poor functional status. MIPPs, indeed, are alternative to conventional surgical interventions for patients who are not

© Springer International Publishing Switzerland 2016
M. Cascella et al., *Features and Management of the Pelvic Cancer Pain*, DOI 10.1007/978-3-319-33587-2_9

good candidates for surgery, as well as in clinical situations in which other approaches—like sympathetic blocks or spinal analgesia—are ineffective or contraindicated. For instance, treatment with EBRT is the standard of care for patients with localized bone pain, with an excellent palliation in the majority of these patients; however, many patients do not experience pain relief with both single and multiple fractions, so it is necessary for a retreatment [5] or the use of other techniques, such as one of MIPPs.

MIPPs play a significant role if there is an identified lesion which is the cause of the painful syndrome. The lesion to be treated may be a primitive pelvic cancer, such as prostate cancer [e.g., through RFA, irreversible electroporation (IRE), or cryoablation] or malignant melanoma of the skin, anus, or vagina [e.g., through electrochemotherapy (ECT)]. Moreover, MIPPs can be successfully used to treat local recurrence or pelvic metastasis. For this purpose, these treatments should be considered as first choice in recurrent pelvic lesions after resection of colorectal cancer and in well-defined metastasis, if the patient is not eligible for a surgical resection. For this purpose, Ohhigashi et al. reported two cases of RFA in recurrence of rectal cancer [6], and this procedure improved QoL providing pain relief for long time [7].

Painful osteolytic bone metastasis of the pelvis represents an important field of application of some MIPPs, such as RFA and percutaneous cryoablation. This is a key point in palliation of cancer pain, as the presence of bone metastases is the most common cause of cancer-related pain [8]. According to Müller et al. [9], patients with multiple osteoblastic lesions at any site and osteolytic or mixed lesions in non-weight-bearing bones should be treated through conservative approaches, including chemotherapy, hormonal therapy, and/or irradiation according to the diagnosis. However, they also stated that percutaneous treatments should be considered if the patient has pain not controllable by opioids or not responding to noninvasive therapies, such as external irradiation. This observation was confirmed by a multicenter study which showed a clinical significant pain reduction in painful metastases involving bone [10].

Additionally, these techniques are applicable even in the absence of a precise lesion to perform neurolysis. For instance, cryoneurolysis—also known as cryoanalgesia or cryoneuroablation—is an effective method of peripheral nerve destruction. Thus, it is applicable for craniofacial pain secondary to trigeminal neuralgia and for chest pain due to post-thoracotomy neuromas and post-herpetic neuralgia [11]. Cryoanalgesia is also used to treat no-cancer pelvic pain secondary to neuralgia [12]; nevertheless, there are few data on its application for palliation of pelvic cancer pain. On the other hand, the use of MIPPs is strongly indicated in early phases of pain management as pain control by conventional methods is difficult because high-dose opioids applied through oral, parenteral, or neuroaxillary techniques are contraindicated or result in uncontrollable and severe side effects.

These nonsurgical approaches also have potential drawbacks. Although uncommon, risks may include increased pain, infection, bleeding, and visceral injury. In the absence of accurate data on complications of MIPPs when used in pelvis, we may refer to the overall complications of these procedures. For instance, complications and risk factors for major complications (e.g., advanced patient age, increased tumor size, increased number of applicators) after percutaneous ablation for small renal masses have been well studied [13]. At the same time, Chen and colleagues did not find significant differences in rates of complications or admission between cryoablation and radiofrequency ablation when used for percutaneous renal tumor treatment. They reported 5 % of complications, mostly related to hemorrhage, and 1 % of short-term readmission due to pulmonary embolism and acute-on-chronic kidney injury [14]. In other sites, in a study on the use of ECT in the head and neck region, the authors reported one nearly lethal bleeding, two cases of osteoradionecrosis, and a fistula [15]. Also, irreversible electroporation seems relatively safe without major complications; however, according to Scheffer and co-authors, complications after pancreatic irreversible electroporation appear more severe [16]. In the study on microwave coagulation for palliation of pelvic recurrence of rectal cancer, the authors observed skin necrosis and nerve injury as adverse events; however, they stated that the procedure was safe [17]. These complications affect the skin and peripheral nerves. Atwell and coauthors reported a rate of skin burns following percutaneous renal RFA up to 1 % [18]. These cutaneous lesions occur for improper dispersion of the thermal energy; nevertheless, they often do not require complex interventions. Among the complications, a more important role is played by the nerve injuries, as the neuroanatomy of pelvis is very complex, including nerves that come from the lumbosacral plexus, coccygeal plexus, and pelvic autonomic nerves. Thus, several nerves, most of which are not visible despite imaging guidance, are at risk of injury during percutaneous ablation. Sensory nerve injury may manifest as pain, anesthesia, or paresthesias in specific dermatomal or sensory nerve distributions. There are no reliable data to determine the procedure with less risk for nerve damage in pelvis; however, in renal masses ablation, nerve injury is more often reported following RFA than cryoablation, occurring in 1–6 % of procedures [19].

Summarizing, spinal analgesia and in selected cases, neurolytic sympathetic blocks remain the mainstay in management of pelvic cancer pain intractable and unresponsive to oral or parenteral opioids. Moreover, although palliative RT is the standard of care for patients with pain due to focal metastatic bone lesions, with an excellent palliation in the majority of these patients, MIPPs may be an alternative treatment for palliation of painful metastatic lesions that are resistant to radiation and in cases where further RT is not possible because of limitations of dose to normal structures. It is also possible that MIPPs may play an adjunctive role to the use of RT for palliation of painful metastatic lesions, also in pelvis.

Thus, MIPPs can be a valid therapeutic approach:

- If there is an identified lesion (organ lesion, recurrence, or metastasis) which is the cause of the painful syndrome
- In painful metastases involving bone, especially when resistant to radiation and in cases where RT and/or surgery are contraindicated or not suitable
- For peripheral nerve destruction or other neurolysis (e.g., cryoneuroablation or RFA of Ganglion Impar).

This approach is also justified in early phases of pain management, as pain control by conventional methods is difficult, or in specific clinical condition, such as well-defined cutaneous/subcutaneous nodules by melanoma or metastasis.

Despite the evidence of effectiveness and safety of these interventions, there are still many barriers to accessing MIPPs, including the availability of trained staff, the lack of precise criteria of indication, and the high costs of these techniques [20].

In the literature, described procedures are the radiofrequency ablation, laser-induced interstitial thermotherapy, percutaneous cryoablation, irreversible electroporation, electrochemotherapy, microwave ablation, and cementoplasty. Additionally, midline myelotomy and ultrasound-guided high intensity focused ultrasound ablation are also applicable.

For all these approaches, the main requirement is that the targeted lesions must be sufficiently separated from the central nervous system, major peripheral motor nerves, and critical structures such as bowel and bladder.

9.1 Radiofrequency Ablation

Percutaneous RFA is a form of high temperature thermal therapy that utilizes a high-frequency alternating current that is passed from the needle electrode into the surrounding tissue, resulting in coagulation necrosis by heating tissue to temperatures near 100 °C which is commonly used to treat painful neurologic and bone lesions. It has been studied for the treatment of hepatocellular carcinoma and liver metastasis, and for lung cancer [21] also for palliation in painful rib metastasis due to non-small cell lung cancer [22]. While the first reported use of RFA in the musculoskeletal system was for the treatment of osteoid osteoma [23], this minimally invasive procedure is often used for the palliation of painful osteolytic bone metastasis [24]. In pelvis, RFA can be performed on coccyx, sacrum areas, or by placing a needle electrode directly into the cancer lesion. About the effectiveness of RFA used to treat bone lesions, palliation depends on

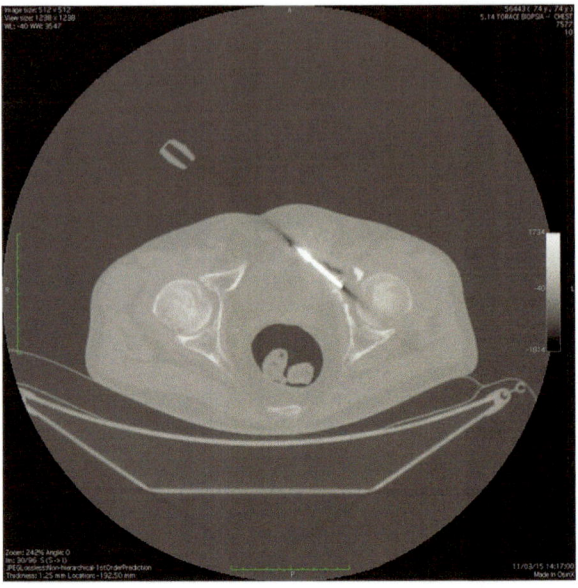

FIGURE 9.1. CT-guided percutaneous radiofrequency ablation of a pelvic bone metastasis (*Courtesy from Prof. F. Fiore. National Cancer Institute, Naples, Italy*)

adequate coverage of the bone–tumor interface, rather than de-bulking the entire tumor (Fig. 9.1) [25]. RFA can be also performed to ablate the Ganglion Impar [26].

9.2   Laser-Induced Thermotherapy

Laser-induced interstitial thermotherapy (LITT), also referred to as percutaneous laser ablation (PLA), is a percutaneous technique in which tissue destruction is induced by a local increase of temperature by means of laser light energy transmission. Moreover, as this technique is often performed by magnetic resonance compatible devices, the incorporation of magnetic resonance imaging for treatment planning and verification has helped to expand the number of applications in which LITT can be applied safely and effectively [27]. This approach was used to treat brain tumors, pulmonary neoplasms, osteoid osteoma, and liver tumors. In pelvis, the technique has been successfully applied for clinically low-risk prostate cancer [28] and for prostate cancer recurrence in the postsurgical prostate bed [29]. For the palliative treatment of spinal metastases, only few cases are reported with a pain relief of maximal 45 % after 3 months [30].

9.3 Percutaneous Cryoablation

In this technique, freezing temperatures induce coagulation necrosis of tissue through several mechanisms of cell death, including direct cell injury due to crystallization of water molecules and interruption of the local microcirculation in the treated tissue zone. The rapid freezing adjacent to the probe results in osmotic differences inducing apoptosis in the periphery of the lesion [31].

Although a minimum cellular temperature of -20 °C appears necessary to provide this effect, this process can result in rapid cooling that reaches -100 °C within a few seconds. Cryoablation has several applications, like hepatocellular carcinoma [32], kidney cancer as alternative to laparoscopic cryoablation [33], malignant lung nodules [34], prostate, and it is considered as primary treatment for small benign bony lesions like osteoid osteoma.

Cryoablation has the important advantage of allowing therapy monitoring because the ice ball that develops can be seen as a well-marginated low-attenuation region on CT or a low-signal region on MR imaging. Moreover, unlike RFA, it does not result in a transient increase in pain after treatment [25]. Consequently, this approach has emerged as a minimally invasive technique for the management of osseous metastases, also in pelvis [35] and leading experts in these techniques stated that the use of cryoablation compared with RFA for palliation of painful metastatic disease involving bone is associated with a greater reduction in analgesic doses and shorter hospital stays after the procedure [36]. Cryoablation has also a role as specialized technique for providing long-term pain relief (cryoanalgesia); indeed, Bellini et al. described the use of percutaneous cryoablation in a case series of 18 patients with articular lumbar facet pain, knee pain, and sacroiliac pain [37].

9.4   Irreversible Electroporation

IRE is a nonthermal form of tissue ablation using high voltage (2–3 kV) direct current. These repeated electrical pulses lasting microseconds to milliseconds induce pores in the lipid bilayer of cells and result in apoptosis without affecting extracellular matrix. Preclinical studies have suggested that IRE may have advantages over conventional forms of thermal tumor ablation including no heat sink effect and preservation of the acellular elements of tissue, resulting in less unwanted collateral damage [38]. Although IRE was used mainly in liver and pancreatic cancer diseases [39], there are some attempts in prostate cancer [40] and in bone metastases in animal models [41].

9.5   Electrochemotherapy

Electrochemotherapy (ECT) is the combined effect of electroporation and the administration of anticancer drugs to treat cancer [42]. Using electric pulses, chemotherapeutic agents, like bleomycin, can enter the tumor cells and accumulates intracellularly. The objective response rate following a single session of treatment exceeds 80 %, with minimal toxicity for the patients. Early evidence suggests that treatment of tumor nodules with ECT recruits components of the immune system and eliciting a systemic immune response against cancer. As this technique is used to treat cutaneous and subcutaneous metastatic tumor nodules, some authors tried it in malignant melanoma of the vagina [43] and in experimental bone metastases in rats [44].

9.6   Microwave Ablation

Microwave energy is used to create localized dielectric heating in order to induce the solidification of proteins in tumor cells and necrosis. In more detail, microwave ablation utilizes an antenna to locally deliver a high frequency (915 MHz or 2.45 GHz) oscillating electromagnetic field to induce rapid realignment of polar molecules (typically water molecules) in a lesion. This results in markedly increased kinetic energy and subsequent tissue heating. Tissues with a larger concentration of water, such as tumors, are particularly susceptible to microwave heating. The microwave ablation has several applications in oncology, for instance, for liver cancer [45]. However, also microwave coagulation therapy for pelvis recurrence or metastasis and pain management needs additional studies. Shimizu et al. treated five recurrent pelvic lesions after curative resection of rectal cancer with magnetic resonance-guided percutaneous microwave coagulation therapy to reduce tumor volume and for pain management [17].

9.7   Cementoplasty and Other Interventions

Bone pelvis metastasis can be managed by cementoplasty which refers to the instillation of polymethylmethacrylate cement into bone. In pelvic painful lesions of the acetabulum or in those involving the bone pelvis, these approaches may result in significant pain relief at 3 days, 1 month, and 3 months postoperatively, with a few rates of complications (cement leakage 12.3 %) [46]. Cementoplasty can also be used as an adjuvant therapy and for this purpose it is commonly performed the day following RFA or cryoablation; indeed, the coagulative necrosis resulting from thermal ablation allows more even distribution of the cement, which then helps to stabilizes weight-bearing bone by sealing microfractures, decreasing the risk of fractures [47, 48]. This combined minimally invasive approach could be also used for symptomatic acetabular lesions (usually treated with surgery), if the patient is not eligible for a more invasive intervention. However, percutaneous treatment is sometimes hampered by technical and anatomical difficulties [49]. Recently, a palliative percutaneous acetabular RFA combined with cementoplasty performed from an anterior approach using a navigational ablation probe and ultrahigh viscosity cement instilled under CT-fluoroscopic guidance has been described [50].

First described by Nauta, midline myelotomy consists of a 5-mm deep puncture using a 16-G needle on either side of the median septum in the dorsal column of the spinal cord (T4, T6, T8, or T10) [51]. The puncture is performed with the intent of interrupting only the midline posterior column visceral pain pathway that ascends to higher brain centers through the midline of the dorsal column. There are few data in literature to judge about the validity and safety of this procedure [52, 53].

Another possible minimally invasive procedure is the ultrasound-guided high intensity focused ultrasound ablation. This technique causes coagulative necrosis of the lesion and it has been used not only to treat uterine submucosal fibroids [54] and liver metastasis [55] but also for palliation of primary malignant neoplasms of the bony pelvis [56]. The procedure appears to be a safe MIPP; however, further studies are warranted to observe its effectiveness.

References

1. Chu L, Hawley P, Munk P et al (2015) Minimally invasive palliative procedures in oncology: a review of a multidisciplinary collaboration. Support Care Cancer 23(6):1589–1596
2. Markmiller M (2015) Percutaneous balloon kyphoplasty of malignant lesions of the spine: a prospective consecutive study in 115 patients. Eur Spine J 24(10):2165–2172
3. Loev MA, Varklet VL, Wilsey BL et al (1988) Cryoablation: a novel approach to neurolysis of the ganglion Impar. Anesthesiology 88:1391–1393
4. Gürses E (2014) Impar ganglion radiofrequency application in successful management of oncologic perineal pain. J Pak Med Assoc 64(6):697–699

5. Chow E, Zeng L, Salvo N et al (2012) Update on the systematic review of palliative radiotherapy trials for bone metastases. Clin Oncol (R Coll Radiol) 24(2):112–124

6. Ohhigashi S, Nishio T, Watanabe F et al (2001) Experience with radiofrequency ablation in the treatment of pelvic recurrence in rectal cancer: report of two cases. Dis Colon Rectum 44:741–745

7. Campos FG, Habr-Gama A, Kiss DR et al (2005) Management of the pelvic recurrence of rectal cancer with radiofrequency thermoablation: a case report and review of the literature. Int J Colorectal Dis 20(1):62–66

8. Mercadante S (1997) Malignant bone pain: pathophysiology and treatment. Pain 69(1–2):1–18

9. Müller DA, Capanna R (2015) The surgical treatment of pelvic bone metastases. Adv Orthop 2015:525363. doi:10.1155/2015/525363

10. Goetz MP, Callstrom MR, Charboneau JW et al (2004) Percutaneous image-guided radiofrequency ablation of painful metastases involving bone: a multicenter study. J Clin Oncol 22(2):300–306

11. Trescot AM (2003) Cryoanalgesia in interventional pain management. Pain Physician 6(3):345–360

12. Peng PW, Tumber PS (2008) Ultrasound-guided interventional procedures for patients with chronic pelvic pain—a description of techniques and review of literature. Pain Physician 11(2):215–224

13. Kurup AN (2014) Percutaneous ablation for small renal masses—complications. Semin Intervent Radiol 31(1):42–49

14. Chen JX, Guzzo TJ, Malkowicz SB et al (2015) Complication and readmission rates following same-day discharge after percutaneous renal tumor ablation. J Vasc Interv Radiol 27(1):80–86. doi:10.1016/j.jvir.2015.09.007

15. Landström FJ, Reizenstein JA, Nilsson CO et al (2015) Electrochemotherapy—possible benefits and limitations to its use in the head and neck region. Acta Otolaryngol 135(1):90–95

16. Scheffer HJ, Nielsen K, de Jong MC et al (2014) Irreversible electroporation for nonthermal tumor ablation in the clinical setting: a systematic review of safety and efficacy. J Vasc Interv Radiol 25(7):997–1011

17. Shimizu T, Endo Y, Mekata E et al (2010) Real-time magnetic resonance-guided microwave coagulation therapy for pelvic recurrence of rectal cancer: initial clinical experience using a 0.5 T open magnetic resonance system. Dis Colon Rectum 53(11):1555–1562

18. Atwell TD, Carter RE, Schmit GD et al (2012) Complications following 573 percutaneous renal radiofrequency and cryoablation procedures. J Vasc Interv Radiol 23(1):48–54

19. Gervais DA, McGovern FJ, Arellano RS et al (2005) Radiofrequency ablation of renal cell carcinoma: part 1, indications, results, and role in patient management over a 6-year period and ablation of 100 tumors. AJR Am J Roentgenol 185(1):64–71

20. Bang HJ, Littrup PJ, Goodrich DJ et al (2012) Percutaneous cryoablation of metastatic renal cell carcinoma for local tumor control: feasibility, outcomes, and estimated cost-effectiveness for palliation. J Vasc Interv Radiol 23(6):770–777. doi:10.1016/j. jvir.2012.03.002

21. Lanuti M, Sharma A, Digumarthy SR et al (2009) Radiofrequency ablation for treatment of medically inoperable stage I non-small cell lung cancer. J Thorac Cardiovasc Surg 137(1):160–166

22. Hu M, Zhi X, Zhang J (2015) Radiofrequency ablation (RFA) for palliative treatment of painful non-small cell lung cancer (NSCLC) rib metastasis: experience in 12 patients. Thorac Cancer 6(6):761–764

23. Rosenthal DI, Springfield DS, Gebhardt MC et al (1995) Osteoid osteoma: percutaneous radio-frequency ablation. Radiology 197:451–454

24. Guenette JP, Lopez MJ, Kim E et al (2013) Solitary painful osseous metastases: correlation of imaging features with pain palliation after radiofrequency ablation—a multicenter American College of Radiology Imaging Network study. Radiology 268:907–915

25. Tam A, Ahrar K (2007) Palliative interventions for pain in cancer patients. Semin Intervent Radiol 24:419–429

26. Usta B, Gozdemir M, Sert H et al (2010) Fluoroscopically guided ganglion impar block by pulsed radiofrequency for relieving coccydynia. J Pain Symptom Manage 39(6):e1–e2. doi:10.1016/j. jpainsymman.2010.02.005

27. Stafford RJ, Fuentes D, Elliott AA (2010) Laser-induced thermal therapy for tumor ablation. Crit Rev Biomed Eng 38(1):79–100

28. Oto A, Sethi I, Karczmar G et al (2013) MR imaging-guided focal laser ablation for prostate cancer: phase I trial. Radiology 267(3):932–940

29. Woodrum DA, Mynderse LA, Gorny KR (2011) 3.0T MR-guided laser ablation of a prostate cancer recurrence in the postsurgical prostate bed. J Vasc Interv Radiol 22(7):929–934

30. Groenemeyer DHW, Schirp S, Gevargez A (2002) Image-guided percutaneous thermal ablation of bone tumors. Acad Radiol 9(4):467–477

31. Gage AA, Baust JC (2007) Cryosurgery for tumors. J Am Coll Surg 205:342–356

32. Wang C, Wang H, Yang W et al (2015) Multicenter randomized controlled trial of percutaneous cryoablation versus radiofrequency ablation in hepatocellular carcinoma. Hepatology 61(5):1579–1590

33. Rodriguez Faba O, Sanguedolce F, Grange P et al (2015) Kidney cancer focal cryoablation trend: does location or approach matter? World J Urol. doi:10.1007/s00345-015-1716-z

34. Yamauchi Y, Izumi Y, Hashimoto K et al (2012) Percutaneous cryoablation for the treatment of medically inoperable stage I non-small cell lung cancer. PLoS One 7(3), e33223. doi:10.1371/journal.pone.0033223

35. Callstrom MR, Atwell TD, Charboneau JW et al (2006) Painful metastases involving bone: percutaneous image-guided cryoablation—prospective trial interim analysis. Radiology 241(2):572–580

36. Thacker PG, Callstrom MR, Curry TB et al (2011) Palliation of painful metastatic disease involving bone with imaging-guided treatment: comparison of patients' immediate response to radiofrequency ablation and cryoablation. AJR Am J Roentgenol 197(2):510–515

37. Bellini M, Barbieri M (2015) Percutaneous cryoanalgesia in pain management: a case-series. Anaesthesiol Intensive Ther 47(4):333–335

38. Charpentier KP (2012) Irreversible electroporation for the ablation of liver tumors: are we there yet? Arch Surg 147(11):1053–1061

39. Gonzalez-Beicos A, Venkat S, Songrug T et al (2015) Irreversible electroporation of hepatic and pancreatic malignancies: radiologic-pathologic correlation. Tech Vasc Interv Radiol 18(3):176–182

40. Valerio M, Ahmed HU, Emberton M (2015) Focal therapy of prostate cancer using irreversible electroporation. Tech Vasc Interv Radiol 18(3):147–152

41. Tschon M, Salamanna F, Ronchetti M et al (2015) Feasibility of electroporation in bone and in the surrounding clinically relevant structures: a preclinical investigation. Technol Cancer Res Treat. doi:10.1177/1533034615604454

42. Cadossi R, Ronchetti M, Cadossi M (2014) Locally enhanced chemotherapy by electroporation: clinical experiences and perspective of use of electrochemotherapy. Future Oncol 10(5):877–890

43. Gauthier T, Uzan C, Gouy S et al (2012) Mélanome vaginal: une localization particulièrement défavorable. Gynecol Obstet Fertil 40(5):273–278

44. Fini M, Salamanna F, Parrilli A et al (2013) Electrochemotherapy is effective in the treatment of rat bone metastases. Clin Exp Metastasis 30(8):1033–1045

45. Poggi G, Tosoratti N, Montagna B et al (2015) Microwave ablation of hepatocellular carcinoma. World J Hepatol 7(25): 2578–2589

46. Sun G, Jin P, Liu XW et al (2014) Cementoplasty for managing painful bone metastases outside the spine. Eur Radiol 24(3):731–737

47. Sapkota BH, Hirsch AE, Yoo AJ et al (2009) Treatment of metastatic carcinoma to the hip with CT-guided percutaneous acetabuloplasty: report of four cases. J Vasc Interv Radiol 20:548–552

48. Kurup AN, Callstrom MR (2010) Image-guided percutaneous ablation of bone and soft tissue tumors. Semin Intervent Radiol 27(3):276–284. doi:10.1055/s-0030-1261786

49. Bauones S, Freire V, Moser TP (2015) Retrograde transpubic approach for percutaneous radiofrequency ablation and cementoplasty of acetabular metastasis. Case Rep Radiol 2015:146963. doi:10.1155/2015/146963

50. Wallace AN, Huang AJ, Vaswani D et al (2016) Combination acetabular radiofrequency ablation and cementoplasty using a navigational radiofrequency ablation device and ultrahigh viscosity cement: technical note. Skeletal Radiol 45(3):401–405

51. Nauta HJW, Hewitt E, Westlund KN et al (1996) Surgical interruption of a midline dorsal column visceral pain pathway: case report and review of the literature. J Neurosurg 86:538–542

52. Becker R, Gatscher S, Sure U (2002) The punctate midline myelotomy concept for visceral cancer pain control—case report and review of the literature. Acta Neurochir Suppl 79:77–78

53. Hong D, Andrén-Sandberg A (2007) Punctate midline myelotomy: a minimally invasive procedure for the treatment of pain in inextirpable abdominal and pelvic cancer. J Pain Symptom Manage 33(1):99–109

54. Wang W, Wang Y, Wang T et al (2012) Safety and efficacy of US-guided high-intensity focused ultrasound for treatment of submucosal fibroids. Eur Radiol 22(11):2553–2558

55. Rossi M, Raspanti C, Mazza E et al (2013) High-intensity focused ultrasound provides palliation for liver metastasis causing gastric outlet obstruction: case report. J Ther Ultrasound 1:9. doi:10.1186/2050-5736-1-9

56. Wang Y, Wang W, Tang J (2013) Primary malignant tumours of the bony pelvis: US-guided high intensity focused ultrasound ablation. Int J Hyperthermia 29(7):683–687

Chapter 10
Psychological, Behavioral, and Rehabilitation Approaches to Cancer Pain Management

Cancer pain is usually treated medically with pharmacological and non-pharmacological approaches; nevertheless, both patients and healthcare professionals often underestimate the impact of cancer pain on psychological distress and do not consider the potential benefits of psychological treatments to help manage cancer pain. According to Dame Cicely Saunders, cancer pain is a "total pain" because the patient's pain experience has physical, emotional, social, and spiritual dimensions [1].

Furthermore, tumors of the pelvis can have a great psychological impact. For instance, cancers of the cervix raise issues like sexuality, femininity, and social isolation; thus, sexual dysfunction and alteration of the body image often represent a major concern, as well as an important cause of distress among women [2]. In survivors of prostate cancer, overall satisfaction with follow-up care was high, but was lower for psychosocial than physical aspects of care. In a survey, it was found that 17 % of men reported potentially moderate-to-severe levels of anxiety and 10.2 % reported moderate-to-severe levels of depression [3]. Yet, the emotional state of patients with permanent colostomy is typically characterized by fear and worry about their current process; indeed, body image, self-esteem, social activity, and sexuality are the aspects that most affect the patients [4]. These are just a few of the many examples. Psychological distress is related to the symptoms of patients with cancer of the pelvis and, consequently,

© Springer International Publishing Switzerland 2016
M. Cascella et al., *Features and Management of the Pelvic Cancer Pain*, DOI 10.1007/978-3-319-33587-2_10

psychological support and care must be integral to the cancer treatment.

According to previous finding, there is a strong linkage between the degree, and the length of the cancer pain experience, and the psychological functioning, especially in terms of negative effect on mood, with anxiety, depressive feelings, and suicidal thoughts [5]. Compared to pain-free cancer patients, cancer patients with pain had significantly higher levels of anxiety, depression, and anger, and patients with higher pain intensity and longer duration of pain had the highest levels of mood disturbance [6]. Several studies showed that social activities, such as visits and conversations, decreased significantly with increasing pain; thus, pain not only causes physical suffering but also influences different aspects of QoL [7], becoming a significant emotional, social, and existential distress [8]. Additionally, and especially in patients with advanced cancer, unrelieved emotions, depressive or anxious symptoms, delirium, and difficulties in communicating greatly influence the expression of pain. While all these findings indicate that in cancer patients psychological factors influence both the experience of pain and the response to pain treatment, psychological and behavioral treatments are not of secondary importance in cancer patient management, and the possibility of reducing psychological distress may improve pain management in any phase of care [9].

There are several psychological and behavioral interventions that can be used in cancer pain management, with cognitive and/or behavioral features. Cognitive behavioral therapy includes a group of interventions teaching patients to respond to pain awareness with a shift in their thoughts and/or coping behaviors. The rationale is that people who experience cancer pain typically develop and use a number of coping strategies to cope with, deal with, or minimize the effects of pain [10]. On this basis, because health professionals should make efforts to understand how each patient copes with pain, also supporting the patient in developing pain coping skills, the presence of a cognitivist psychologist as component of the pain management team is often mandatory. As support of these observations, a meta-analysis concluded that cognitive behavioral therapy techniques have beneficial effects on pain and distress in women with breast cancer, finding moderate effect sizes of drugs used in pain management [11].

Cognitive behavioral therapy may help patients cope with cancer and the psychosocial problems associated with cancer and cancer treatment, but is less likely to help with common physical issues such as loss of strength and flexibility, weight gain, and reduced physical function [12]. Thus, some authors prefer behavioral approaches that are based on behavioral training studied to teach patients the use of adaptive behaviors, like engaging in distracting activities, pacing activities, and appropriate use of medications or physical modalities [13]. Patients may be taught to observe what increases pain and to take a pain medication before that activity, or they may learn when their pain is less severe in a specific moment of the day, in order to do their priority activities during that time. Behavioral approaches are also relaxation, imagery, exercise, or yoga. These treatments provide physiologic benefits, adding competing sensory input to the brain, which can shift thoughts and emotional responses. Yoga, for example, is feasible for patients with cancer, with improved sleep, QoL, mood, and levels of stress [14]. Other strategies, like meditation or hypnosis, shift focus away from pain, also in pediatric patients, in which these therapies have been shown to reduce anticipatory anxiety, procedure-related pain, procedure-related anxiety, and behavioral distress during venipuncture [15]. Educational interventions often include both behavioral approaches and cognitive behavioral therapy elements that provide adaptive coping skills and address barriers to the use of treatments for pain, as well as increase understanding of how to use treatment options and how to communicate with healthcare providers about pain. Other psychosocial methods include a focus on partner/caregiver responses to pain or supportive-expressive or meaning-centered therapies that allow patients to explore their feelings, needs, and interpretation of their experiences with a supportive and facilitating therapist.

Psychologists have also a paramount role in the doctor–patient relationship. In fact, cancer patients should be full partners in decision-making, and the pluses and minuses of each option should be explained and in most instances the patient should have the final call. Nevertheless, physicians may encounter communication difficulties; then the opportunity to receive help from experts is not to be underestimated. For example, probable side effects and complications of treatments must be well known by patients, and yet, in case of invasive procedure, consultation regarding preferred site of catheter exit and implantable pump should also be sought and respected.

Because cancer pain may be due to the cancer itself or secondary to immobility and debilitation, it may benefit from interventions that focus on function. For this purpose, mobility—and consequently pain—may be improved by strengthening, stretching, and the use of assistive devices; thus, including a rehabilitation medicine specialist in the pain management team is often a winning move.

Treatment objectives of cancer rehabilitation are preventive, to improve function and reduce morbidity and disability; restorative, for patients with potential cure of cancer whose residual disability can be appropriately controlled or eliminated; supportive for patients who must continue with cancer but can expect relative control or remission of appreciable time; and palliative.

As well described by Cheville et al. [16], rehabilitative and physical modalities used to manage pain can operate by modulating nociception, stabilizing the painful structures, and influencing physiological processes that indirectly influence nociception. Additionally, these interventions can alleviate pain arising from the overloading of muscles and connective tissues that often occurs after surgery or with sarcopenia in late-stage of the cancer disease. Cancer rehabilitative treatments include physical therapy, occupational therapy, lymphedema therapy, recreational therapy, speech and language pathology therapies, and the use of prosthetics and orthotics. These treatments may be particularly beneficial to patients with movement-associated pain [16] and in some clinical condition, for instance to manage post radiation complications, like neuromuscular and musculoskeletal complications of the radiation fibrosis syndrome [17].

Specific therapies, such as occupational therapy, can be particularly effective to help pain management in selected cases of cancer patients, also in pelvic neoplastic diseases. The role of occupational therapy in oncology and cancer-related pain management is well recognized today [18]. Occupational therapy is a rehabilitation approach which uses assessment and treatment to develop, recover, or maintain the daily living and work skills of people with a physical, mental, or cognitive disorder. In oncology, it can help patients to continue or resume usual roles despite cancer-related pain; indeed, by this intervention, the patient receives a constructive help to build perceived personal control or self-efficacy to manage cancer pain [19]. Occupational therapy works through interventions on productivity and leisure, self-care—for instance, with the purpose of maintaining or increasing autonomy in performing activities of daily living, or creating an action plan to optimize treatment adherence—cognitive and affective aspects, physical aspect of the person, and spirituality [20]. According to Lapointe, an optimal occupational intervention should be personalized, scilicet well chosen, carefully graded and monitored, and appropriate to the patient's cancer stage [21]. Occupational therapy could be effective in sick cancer patients and in those with cognitive impairments, mental illness, language barriers, or suspected substance abuse. Probably, the odds of having any potentially modifiable functional deficit are higher in patients with increasing age, comorbid conditions, and with less than a college degree [22]. However, as reported by Mackenzie Pergolotti and colleagues, only 32 % of adult patients used occupational therapy within the first 2 years of their cancer diagnosis (also prostate and colorectal cancer), a rate lower than the estimated 87 % who are in need of such approach [23].

For all these considerations, in pelvic cancer pain, the most suitable psychological, behavioral, and rehabilitation approach should be chosen after a case-by-case analysis to improve the QoL and the psychosocial outcomes, the compliance to the therapy, and the doctor–patient interaction/relationship.

Messages for the Head of the Pain Management Team

- Tumors of the pelvis can have a great psychological impact.
- Many evidences underline the effective role of psychological, behavioral, and rehabilitation approaches to cancer-related pain.
- Include specialists in those fields within the interdisciplinary pain team management.

References

1. Richmond C (2005) Obituary: Dame Cicely Saunders. BMJ 331(7510):238
2. Kulhari P, Ayyagari S, Nehra R (1988) Psychological aspects of cervix cancer. Indian J Psychol Med 11:79–83
3. Watson E, Shinkins B, Frith E et al (2015) Symptoms, unmet needs, psychological well-being and health status in survivors of prostate cancer: implications for redesigning follow-up. BJU Int. doi:10.1111/bju.13122
4. Dabirian A, Yaghmaei F, Rassouli M et al (2011) Quality of life in ostomy patients: a qualitative study. Patient Prefer Adherence 5:1–5
5. Zaza C, Baine N (2002) Cancer pain and psychosocial factors: a critical review of the literature. J Pain Symptom Manage 24:526–542
6. Glover J, Dibble SL, Dodd MF et al (1995) Mood states of oncology patients: does pain make a difference? J Pain Symptom Manage 10:120–128
7. Strang P, Qvarner H (1990) Cancer-related pain and its influence on quality of life. Anticancer Res 10(1):109–112
8. Strang P (1998) Cancer pain—a provoker of emotional, social and existential distress. Acta Oncol 37(7–8):641–644
9. Syrjala KL, Jensen MP, Mendoza ME et al (2014) Psychological and behavioral approaches to cancer pain management. J Clin Oncol 32(16):1703–1711
10. Bishop SR, Warr D (2003) Coping, catastrophizing and chronic pain in breast cancer. J Behav Med 26:265–281

11. Tatrow K, Montgomery GH (2006) Cognitive behavioral therapy techniques for distress and pain in breast cancer patients: a meta-analysis. J Behav Med 29:17–27
12. Emslie C, Whyte F, Campbell A et al (2007) 'I wouldn't have been interested in just sitting round a table talking about cancer'; exploring the experiences of women with breast cancer in a group exercise trial. Health Educ Res 22:827–838
13. Buffart LM, van Uffelen JG, Riphagen II et al (2012) Physical and psychosocial benefits of yoga in cancer patients and survivors, a systematic review and meta-analysis of randomized controlled trials. BMC Cancer 12:559. doi:10.1186/1471-2407-12-559
14. Lin K-Y, Hu Y-T, Chang K-J et al (2011) Effects of yoga on psychological health, quality of life, and physical health of patients with cancer: a meta-analysis. Evid Based Complement Alternat Med 2011:659876. doi:10.1155/2011/659876
15. Montgomery GH, Schnur JB, Kravits K (2013) Hypnosis for cancer care: over 200 years young. CA Cancer J Clin 63:31–44
16. Cheville AL, Basford JR (2014) Role of rehabilitation medicine and physical agents in the treatment of cancer-associated pain. J Clin Oncol 32(16):1691–1702
17. Stubblefield MD (2009) Radiation fibrosis syndrome. In: Stubblefield MD, O'Dell MW (eds) Cancer rehabilitation: principles and practice. Demos Medical Publishing, New York, pp 723–745
18. Bloch R (2004) Rehabilitation medicine approach to cancer pain. Cancer Invest 22(6):944–948
19. Bandura A (1977) Self-efficacy: toward a unifying theory of behavioral change. Psychol Rev 84(2):191–215
20. Lloyd C, Coggles L (1988) Contribution of occupational therapy to pain management in cancer patient with metastatic breast disease. Am J Hosp Care 5(6):36–38
21. Lapointe J (2012) Cancer-related pain: the role of occupational therapy in prevention and management. OccupTher Now 14(5):10–12
22. Pergolotti M, Deal AM, Lavery J (2015) The prevalence of potentially modifiable functional deficits and the subsequent use of occupational and physical therapy by older adults with cancer. J Geriatr Oncol 6(3):194–201
23. Pergolotti M, Cutchin MP, Weinberger M et al (2014) Occupational therapy use by older adults with cancer. Am J Occup Ther 68(5):597–607

Chapter 11
Pain Management Team and Palliative Care Setting

Approximately, 65 % of persons diagnosed with cancer today can expect to live at least 5 years after diagnosis compared with only 35 % in the 1950s and 50 % in the 1980s [1]. There are more than 13 million cancer survivors in the USA today, and the number will likely increase to 18 million by 2022 [2]. More than half of these patients are survivors of abdominal or pelvic cancers. This evidence suggests the need to be able to assist a growing number of cancer survivor patients.

No recent studies have already shown improved outcomes from using specialist and multidisciplinary pain management services [3]. In many cases, multidisciplinary approach focused on providing patients with relief from the symptoms, like pain, or physical and mental stress (e.g., fatigue) and follows a parallel course with the diagnosis and the pharmacological and non-pharmacological management of the cancer disease. In this eventuality, pain management, combined with all the treatments used to manage side effects of cancer therapies, plays a fundamental role to ensure a good QoL for both the patient and the family.

In the course of disease, pain management works in conjunction with other therapies that are intended to prolong life, such as chemotherapy or RT, and includes those investigations needed to better understand and manage distressing clinical complications. However, a modern pain treatment is never focused on just the pain, but it takes a holistic approach to the patient and his disease, and his family, offering a complete

© Springer International Publishing Switzerland 2016   151
M. Cascella et al., *Features and Management of the Pelvic Cancer Pain*, DOI 10.1007/978-3-319-33587-2_11

program from assessment, treatment, communication, education, and follow up, such as fatigue, loss of appetite, nausea, vomiting, shortness of breath, and insomnia. Moreover, an effective cancer pain management needs to be client centered and family members or friends are important allies to consider in this context.

Assuming that the concept of team refers to a way of being, of thinking, and to collaborative and interactive work, a more correct approach to pain control should be provided by a multidisciplinary team under the responsibility of a pain specialist coordinating several professionals to create an individualized care plan. Consequently, the pain management should begin at diagnosis and continue through treatment and follow-up care, until the end of life [4].

Specialist clinicians involved in the management of pelvic cancer pain include pain specialists (usually the team head), oncologists, neurologists [5], rheumatologists [6], radiation therapists, orthopedic surgeons (e.g., for management of pelvic bone metastasis), surgeons (e.g., for management of recurrence or cancer complications, such as fistula), and psychiatrists. Usually, the head of the pain management team is a pain specialist: an expert in assessing and treating pain. Nevertheless, different specialists, such as anesthesiologists, may also have an additional specialization in pain management, and their expertise is needful to deliver advanced pain management procedures ranging from peripheral or central nerve blocks to device implantation and other procedures like MIPPs. Anesthesiologists have much experience using potent analgesic drugs as well as surgical or neural blockade, and in some countries, for example, the UK and Italy, anesthesia is the only specialty that incorporates advanced pain management within its training program. The clinical nurse specialist is a key figure in the team, as he/she is involved in educating patients about health conditions and their treatment, prevention and health maximization activities, clinical procedures and surgery, and other patient care as advised by the treating doctor. Also physiotherapists, occupational therapists, rehabilitation counselors, psychologists, social workers, and volunteers are involved. Additionally, other medical specialists such as pediatricians, surgical oncologists, and neurosurgeons participate when pain associated with the disease may require their expertise. A gynecologist or an urologist may be included in the core team for the management of patients with pelvic cancer pain.

When no cure of the cancer disease can be expected, pain management becomes an important component of the palliative care setting. Palliative care, also called comfort care, supportive care, and symptom management, refers to active, global, and multidisciplinary care of patients with oncological or non-oncological pain which does not respond to specific treatments. The aim is to assist the patient during the last stage of his/her life. The most noticeable benefit of palliative care is the relief of physical symptoms such as pain, fatigue, lack of appetite, nausea and vomiting, or shortness of breath. Relief from pain is one among the main targets of palliative care, and also in this care setting opioids are the drugs of first choice for severe and moderately severe cancer-related pain and for breathlessness [7].

According to the WHO definition, this approach has the aim to improve the QoL of patients and their families facing the problem associated with life-threatening illness, through the prevention and relief of suffering by means of early identification and impeccable assessment and treatment of pain and other problems, physical, psychosocial, and spiritual [8]. The key point is that palliative care intends neither to hasten nor postpone death and at the same time affirms life and regards dying as a normal process. This approach often represents an ideal model because many patients experience severe, unnecessary symptoms during treatment as well as at the end of life, and others receive "aggressive" care that is discordant with their preferences [9].

The palliative approaches can be delivered in hospitals, institutions predominantly specialized in providing care in an end of life, or at home; nevertheless, evidence of benefit, in terms of end-of-life experiences of patients and their caregivers, is strongest for the home care setting [10].

In regard to the timing for starting the palliative care setting, it is evident that this approach is frequently misconstrued as synonymous with end-of-life care. However, substantial evidence demonstrates that palliative care, when combined with standard cancer care or as the main focus of care, leads to better patient and caregiver outcomes [11], with significant improvements in both QoL and mood [12]. Consequently, this piece of data should lead to integrating palliative care services into standard oncology practice at the time a person is diagnosed with metastatic or advanced cancer [13].

Because of the lack of a precise outcome, it could be difficult to determine the efficacy of a palliative care program. A systematic review on satisfaction with care at the end of life showed that different types of palliative care interventions can improve satisfaction [14] which can be understood as the sum of several domains, as accessibility and coordination; competence, including symptom management; communication and education; emotional support and personalization of care; and support of patients' decision-making.

The members of a palliative care team have specific and multifactorial features; they respond not only to medical but also psychological and social needs of the patients; and they should have sympathy, moderation, communication, and reassurance skills. In general, the interdisciplinary palliative care team is more complex than the pain management team, with a prevalent interest in pain management and emotional and psychological support. Basically, it includes a doctor, a nurse, and a social worker, but other experts often complete the team, according to a patient's needs. Also, a palliative team may include surgeons, interventional radiologists, radiotherapists, and oncologists; however, the role of pharmacists, dieticians, nurses, rehabilitation specialists, and physical therapists is more important for the purpose of care setting. There is no single model for a palliative care team, so other professional roles can participate to integrate the psychological and spiritual aspects of patient care, such as chaplains, counselors, music and art therapists, and home health aides. There may be a benefit of music therapy on the QoL of people in end-of-life care [15], while also psychotherapy has an important role in the palliative care setting, with interventions which can be delivered to the patients alone, to caregivers alone, or to the family system. Psychotherapy can be provided in conjunction with psychotropic medications to relieve symptoms such as anxiety and depression or alone when medications are contraindicated or patients prefer to address their distress in non-pharmacological ways [16]. Nevertheless, the goal of the psychotherapy in palliative care setting is to deliver an aid for both patients and caregivers to improve coping and reduce the suffering resulting from the awareness that death may be near. Moreover, it can also be used effectively to improve communication between patients and other members of the treatment team.

Suggestions for Palliative Care Setting

- Also in palliative care setting, opioids are the drugs of first choice for severe and moderately severe cancer-related pain and for breathlessness.
- Use medication to prevent opioid-related constipation.
- Consider that no clinically relevant opioid-related respiratory depression was observed in any study.
- Consider that pain and fatigue are strongly positively correlated.
- Address the emotional and spiritual concerns and those of the caregivers.
- Together with pain and breathlessness, another relatively frequent symptom in the dying phase is delirium. Treatment with haloperidol is recommended.
- Anxiety and depression should be treated with antidepressant and benzodiazepines, but consider that psychotherapy is also effective for this purpose, even in patients with a short life expectancy.
- Because palliative care intends neither to hasten nor postpone death, when the dying phase begins, tumor-specific treatments should be stopped.

References

1. Howlader N, Noone AM, Krapcho M et al (2014) SEER Cancer Statistics Review, 1975–2012. National Cancer Institute. http://seer.cancer.gov/csr/1975_2012/, based on November 2014 SEER data submission, posted to the SEER web site, April 2015

2. Siegel R, DeSantis C, Virgo K et al (2012) Cancer treatment and survivorship statistics. CA Cancer J Clin 62(4):220–241

3. Banning A, Sjogren P, Henriksen H (1991) Treatment outcome in a multidisciplinary cancer pain clinic. Pain 47(2):129–134

4. Bausewein C, Simon ST, Pralong A et al (2015) Palliative care of adult patients with cancer. Dtsch Arztebl Int 112(50):863–870

5. Lalani I (2006) Emerging subspecialities in neurology: pain medicine. Neurology 67(8):1522–1523

6. Cooper RG, Booker CK, Spanswick CC (2003) What is pain management, and what is its relevance to the rheumatologist? Rheumatology 42(10):1133–1137

7. Chwistek M, Ewerth N (2016) Opioids and chronic pain in cancer survivors: evolving practice for palliative care clinics. J Palliat Med 19(3):254. doi:10.1089/jpm.2015.0471

8. WHO (2009) Definition of palliative care. http://www.who.int/cancer/palliative/definition/en/. Accessed Sept 2015

9. Rocque GB, Cleary JF (2013) Palliative care reduces morbidity and mortality in cancer. Nat Rev Clin Oncol 10(2):80–89

10. Higginson IJ, Finlay IG, Goodwin DM et al (2003) Is there evidence that palliative care teams alter end-of-life experiences of patients and their caregivers? J Pain Symptom Manage 25(2):150–168

11. Nieder C, Norum J (2012) Early palliative care in patients with metastatic non-small cell lung cancer. Ann Palliat Med 1(1):84–86

12. Temel JS, Greer JA, Muzikansky A et al (2010) Early palliative care for patients with metastatic non-small-cell lung cancer. N Engl J Med 363:733–742

13. Smith TJ, Temin S, Alesi ER et al (2012) American Society of Clinical Oncology provisional clinical opinion: the integration of palliative care into standard oncology care. J Clin Oncol 30(8):880–887

14. Dy SM, Shugarman LR, Lorenz KA et al; RAND-Southern California Evidence-Based Practice Center (2008) A systematic review of satisfaction with care at the end of life. J Am Geriatr Soc 56(1):124–129

15. Bradt J, Dileo C (2010) Music therapy for end-of-life care. Cochrane Database Syst Rev 1, CD007169. doi:10.1002/14651858. CD007169.pub2
16. Sheard T, Maguire P (1999) The effect of psychological interventions on anxiety and depression in cancer patients: results of two meta-analyses. Br J Cancer 80(11):1770–1780

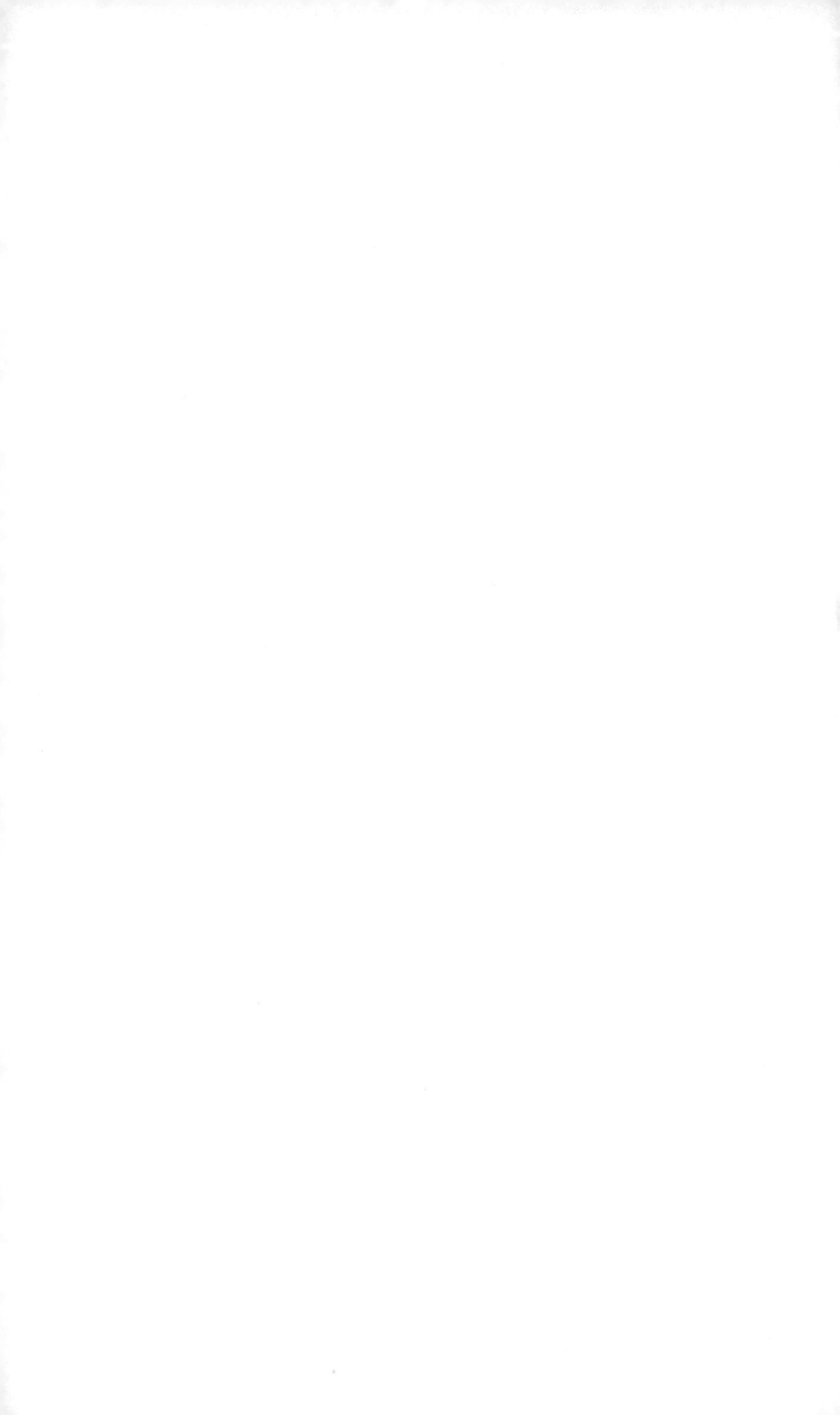

Chapter 12
Conclusion

Cancer-associated pain in advanced neoplastic diseases of the pelvis is often the most debilitating aspect of the malignant disease; therefore, it is recognized as a significant health issue. About 75 % of the patients with pelvic cancer will present pain at any time during disease, and 50 % and 30 % of them will have moderately severe and very severe pain, respectively [1]. Thus, pain management is vital to reduce patients' suffering and improve their overall comfort. However, in contrast with the recommendation of the Declaration of Montréal stating that access to pain management is a fundamental human right [2], this enormous need remains largely unmet [3].

Because of the complex nature of pelvic cancer pain, it is unrealistic to expect one profession or group of specialists to undertake the enormous task of pain management in this setting of patients. Pharmacological management remains the most common method of treating [4]; however, in selected cases, an invasive, or minimally invasive, technique can be preferred in early phases of pain management. The right choice can be difficult, so a correct approach to pelvic cancer pain control should be provided by a multidisciplinary team under the responsibility of a pain specialist coordinating several professionals such as surgeons, interventional radiologists, radiotherapists, and oncologists. This is a big challenge because appropriate use of available therapies can effectively relieve pain in most patients, improving their QoL throughout all stages of the disease.

© Springer International Publishing Switzerland 2016   159
M. Cascella et al., *Features and Management of the Pelvic
Cancer Pain*, DOI 10.1007/978-3-319-33587-2_12

References

1. Portenoy RK (1989) Cancer pain. Epidemiology and syndromes. Cancer 63:2298–2307
2. International Pain Summit Of The International Association For The Study Of Pain (2011) Declaration of Montréal: declaration that access to pain management is a fundamental human right. J Pain Palliat Care Pharmacother 25(1):29–31
3. Weiss SC, Emanuel LL, Fairclough DL et al (2001) Understanding the experience of pain in terminally ill patients. Lancet 357(9265):1311–1315
4. Zekry HA, Reddy SK (1999) Opioid and nonopioid therapy in cancer pain: the traditional and the new. Curr Rev Pain 3:237–247

Appendix A
General Prerequisites and Contraindications Applicable to Interventions (Chaps. 7–9)

In this appendix, both general prerequisites and contraindications applicable to all interventions suitable for pelvic cancer pain management, including Central Neuraxial Blocks, Neurolytic Sympathetic Plexus Blocks, and Minimally Invasive Palliative Treatments, are schematically reported, while considerations regarding the single approaches have been discussed within the specific chapters.

Many of these skills require close cooperation between the various pain team members. For example, in case of bone metastases, choosing the right treatment is a tough challenge, so it is vital to the preliminary clinical assessment which in turn involves collaboration between oncologists and radiologists, or orthopedic surgeons, while the psychologist plays a key role in making the patient understand the risks and benefits of the procedure, and to assess whether she/he and her/his family are able to follow a home care program.

© Springer International Publishing Switzerland 2016   161
M. Cascella et al., *Features and Management of the Pelvic Cancer Pain*, DOI 10.1007/978-3-319-33587-2

General prerequisites applicable to all the interventions useful for pelvic cancer pain management [1–3]

Patient must have received an optimal trial of analgesics as per WHO analgesic ladder and found to be recalcitrant or developed intolerable side effects limiting their use or dose

A physical examination combined with a detailed clinical assessment must precede interventions (degree of the disease, presence of any neurological deficits, comorbidities, drug allergies)

Review an accurate documentation of pain location, frequency, intensity, and its effect on QoL

Consider patient's ability to lie in particular positions for the duration of intervention

Contraindications to interventions should be sought (*see table ad hoc, below*)

Site-specific inspection at the intended puncture site to rule out any local infection should be performed

Because the patient is often immunocompromised, follow strict aseptic technique and adopt a pre-procedure antibiotic cover

In case of neurolytic block, a diagnostic/prognostic block with local anesthetic to explore effectiveness, associated sensory, and motor deficits should be contemplated before any procedure

Investigations including imaging should be ordered and reviewed (anatomical deviations, tumor compression, needle trajectory)

Consider your experience and familiarity with the said procedure

See a recent coagulation profile

Obtain a written informed consent preferably in patient's own language explaining the goals of the procedure, what to expect, probable side effects, and complications

Consider both financial implications and availability of resources and tools

---

General contraindications to all interventions

Absolute	Relative
Patient refusal	Neutropenia
[a]*Bed sores*	Neurological deficits
Local or systemic infection	
Uncorrected coagulopathy	
(INR > 1.5, platelet count < 50,000)	
Uncooperative patient	
Lack of technical expertise	
Uncertainty regarding the diagnosis	
Allergy to the drugs to be used	

[a]Usually, bed sores are included among relative contraindications for interventions. In pelvic pain management, they may become absolute contraindications because of the proximity with the puncture site; however, these recommendations are less stringent in the case of neuraxial blockade and the choice must be made after a case-by-case analysis

Appendix B
Algorithm for Pelvic Cancer Pain Management

© Springer International Publishing Switzerland 2016 163
M. Cascella et al., *Features and Management of the Pelvic
Cancer Pain*, DOI 10.1007/978-3-319-33587-2

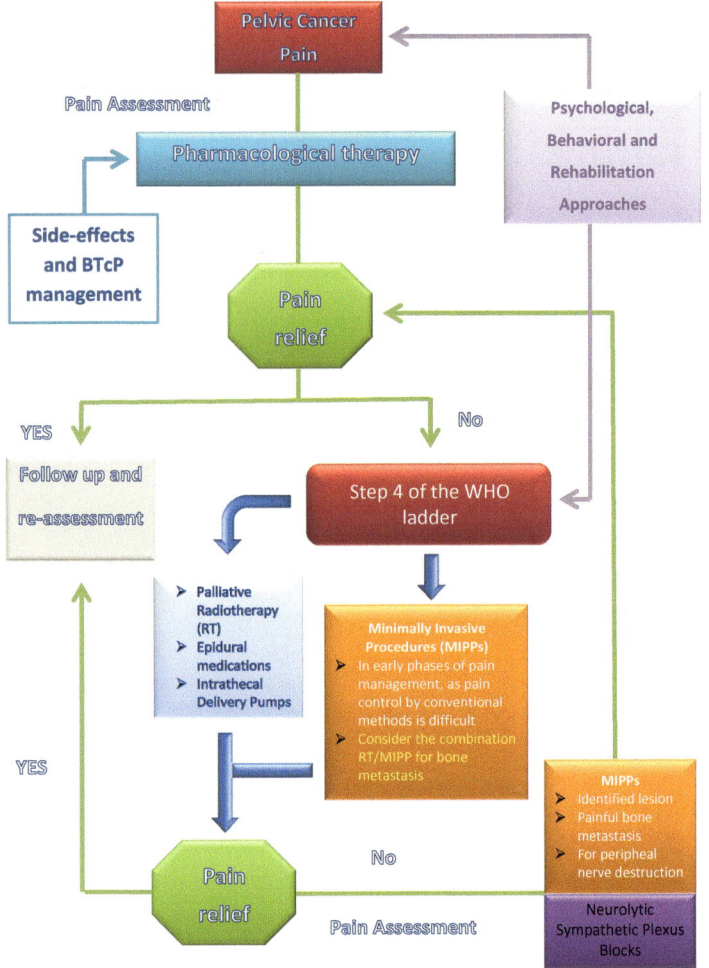